PENITENT, WITH ROSES

The Katharine Bakeless Nason Literary Publication Prizes

The Bakeless Literary Publication Prizes are sponsored by the Bread Loaf Writers' Conference of Middlebury College to support the publication of first books. The manuscripts are selected through an open competition and are published by University Press of New England/Middlebury College Press.

NONFICTION COMPETITION WINNERS

1999
Kevin Oderman, *How Things Fit Together*
judge: Scott Russell Sanders

2000
Paula W. Peterson, *Penitent, with Roses:
An HIV+ Mother Reflects*
judge: Tom Mallon

Penitent, with Roses

An HIV+ Mother Reflects

Paula W. Peterson

MIDDLEBURY COLLEGE PRESS

Published by University Press of New England

Hanover and London

Middlebury College Press

Published by University Press of New England, Hanover, NH 03755

© *2001 by Paula W. Peterson*

All rights reserved

Printed in the United States of America

5 4 3 2 1

"Prognosis Guarded" first appeared in the Spring 1998 issue of *New Millennium Writings*.

Library of Congress Cataloging-in-Publication Data

Peterson, Paula W.
   Penitent, with roses : an HIV+ mother reflects / Paula W. Peterson.
   p. cm.
  ISBN 1–58465–128–8 (alk. paper)
   1. Peterson, Paula W.—Health. 2. AIDS (Disease) in
pregnancy—Patients—California—San Francisco—Biography
3. HIV-positive women—California—San Francisco—Biography.
I. Title.
  RG580.A44 P48 2001
  362.1'969792'0092—dc21   2001002491

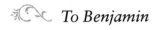 *To Benjamin*

Contents

PENITENT, WITH ROSES

Chapter One

Caesarean

My "pains," as they are so quaintly called, begin in earnest at midnight on November 14, 1995, which happens to be my exact due date. The fact that I am so virtuously on time affords me some solace in the hours ahead, something to hang on to.

We have people over to dinner the evening before, friends of ours and of my parents whose daughter is also expecting a baby shortly, and all throughout the meal I experience periodic contractions. I grasp the edge of the table, stare down at my whitefish swimming in lemon sauce until it passes. The conversation flows around me as if nothing is happening. That is just the way I want it. The important thing is that the evening should continue as planned. And why not? So far the pain is no worse than a bad menstrual cramp.

Yesterday I began passing "brown matter." It is a harbinger of birth—the mucus plug that guarded the opening of the cervix for so many months so that nothing could pass back and forth and disturb the growing fetus has finally loosened. I am both excited and shamed. The brown stuff looks like shit; unlike shit, though, I have no control over it. It simply keeps on coming. I don't know the territory here, like I do with my menstrual period—how many days, how heavy the flow on each day, the menagerie of odors. The "brown matter" follows private rules of its own making.

My husband and I have been saying to each other, "In a few weeks or a few days we're going to have our son." The words are just words, their reality incomprehensible to me—they seem to describe some otherworldly state of being. I am going to be a mother, all right, but there are still some simple rituals to perform in the here and now—saying goodbye to our guests and wishing their daughter well, putting away the leftover food, washing the dishes and tidying up the kitchen, making sure my parents are comfortably bedded down. These are the last few hours that my life will really belong to me. I don't know that, though, and perhaps I don't spend them as I should. Still, these humble tasks are pleasurable. My husband and I turn in early.

At midnight I wake abruptly to find that labor is upon me. No longer is it something I can put aside until I've finished whatever else I am doing. It's like an unwieldy black dog that has climbed into bed with me. With great hope, I commence my breathing.

Who has ever been able to describe the pain of labor? Some women say it feels like riding a wave, or climbing up a steep path. Some say it makes them feel high, spaced out, buzzed, on the edge of a luminous euphoria. Some speak of glaciers and mountains. But these are metaphorical descriptions of the process, not the pain—the pain itself defies all attempts to harness it with words. I could tell you that it was like a thin steel band was tied around your waist and that at first it was just the friction against your skin that caused discomfort, and then, as the hours passed, it was like someone was gradually pulling the band just a little tighter each time, until finally it was grinding deeply into you, past the layers of skin and muscle and tissue, searing every organ of your body and forcing you into a deep well of pain in which you were sure you might drown. And then all of a sudden whoever was tightening the band let go and you went shooting up to the top of the well again gasping for air.

But that won't do it either.

I lie there staring at my husband's immense slumbering back, wondering if I should wake him. He has to go to work the next day. In fact, I am supposed to go to work with him, because his co-workers are going to take us to lunch and present us with a gift. I am looking forward to it. I do not like to be impolite to his co-workers, spoil their plans. And my husband needs his sleep.

A few minutes later I punch him in the side. More urgent forces have usurped politeness. He is difficult to awaken— he shifts, opens his eyes, mumbles, and then goes back to sleep. I have to punch him several times. He says, "It's the middle of the night."

I sit down confidently in a rocking chair. The Lamaze videos showed a woman who endured her entire labor this way, and it is still early enough in this whole process for me to believe this is possible, for me to believe in Lamaze itself.

I breathe faithfully and try to picture myself cresting a small hill, as we had been instructed. I rock. My husband's stop watch reveals that my contractions are three minutes apart. I telephone the hospital.

"Has your bag of waters broken?" the doctor on call asks me.

"No."

"What about blood, any bloody show?"

"No."

"Okay, you're probably not ready. When the pains get worse, then it'll be time to come in."

"Worse—?"

"I know it feels painful to you, but if you came in now, we'd probably examine you and send you right back home. Wait until morning. Try to get some sleep. Or get into a hot bath and soak for awhile. You'll feel better."

I am mortified; I am sorry to have bothered this busy doctor. I lecture myself on my foolishness. I tell myself that next time I will certainly put up with a little discomfort rather than rushing to the phone.

So I go to bed and sleep fitfully until morning. Somehow, I struggle through until noon. The same instincts that propelled me at dinner last night propel me now; I take a shower, wash and blow dry my hair, put on make-up. A contraction hits me as I am applying lipstick, and I draw a red smudge across my cheek. I do not think much about the baby at all. Maybe I figure he can take care of himself, maybe I figure he will forgive me this selfishness, just once. I need all of me for *me* right now.

By noon I have had enough of stoicism. The moment I get into the car to go to the hospital, of course, the pain subsides. The now-familiar shame takes its place, tinged with a peculiar nostalgic longing. It is a beautiful sunny day, and as we drive through the park I see people jogging, mothers with baby strollers (but I avert my eyes from these), bicyclists, old ladies out for a breath of fresh air. I might be out here myself, I think, if it wasn't for this neurosis of mine, this conviction that I am in labor. With my ridiculous swollen belly, my phantom pains, I am making an ass of myself. I have things to do and my parents are here, I certainly don't want to trouble them like this—and it's prime weather, I want to enjoy it—and on and on until I nearly tell my husband to turn around and go home again. Then, a pain doubles me over. Too late! I can never join the joggers and bicyclists now.

* * *

I conceived my baby cavalierly, without trying too hard, although I had thought it would be otherwise. For most of my life I did not think about babies or have any desire for them. In my twenties I harbored a romantic notion that I was "barren." This may have been reinforced by the fact that as a young girl, too thin and too athletic, I often went six months or more without having a period; I had also been on the Pill for many years and had been told by a doctor that the hormonal interference might make conception a lengthier process. And as a writer, I nursed a conviction, quite legitimate, that any fertility I possessed would be manifested through my art, not my body. What could nature do, faced with such an attitude, except outfox me? I got pregnant in lightning speed, like a rabbit or a teenaged girl.

My husband and I could never say to each other definitively, "I want a baby," so, cowards, we made the next best decision: to stop using birth control, and to see what would happen next. The first morning I deliberately did not take the little pink pill, I broke into a panic at the bus stop on the way to work. The bus came; I turned tail and ran home again, swallowed the pill, and caught a later bus. The next month I was more successful at refraining from the Pill. When I got my period, I was relieved. But I found this relief unsettling—I did not need to analyze myself too deeply to understand all the dangerous implications of my ambivalence. I promised myself that at the beginning of my cycle, after I got my next period, I would go back on the Pill. But my next period never came.

My reaction to the home pregnancy test was an outburst of histrionic tears. (The notorious hormones were already having their way with me.) Angrily I declared my mastery over biological laws—why should my body undergo certain processes without my conscious consent? Could it not sense my hesitation? Did not an ovum have a moral obligation to resist fertilization, if the owner of the ovaries was of two minds about conception?

Of course, it was only a few weeks before I became an enthusiastic co-conspirator in biology's ultimatum. I embraced my pregnancy, threw myself wholeheartedly into waistline measurements, morning sickness, urine tests, "how-to" texts, maternity clothes. I wept over a famous Swedish photographer's amazing pictures of embryos at different stages of development; I wept again, hormone-laden, every time I picked up a certain tiny yellow knit sweater, with matching cap and booties.

But until you actually give birth, the baby is all speculation and pregnancy is a game. No matter how difficult the nine months may be (and mine were relatively easy) they cannot prepare you for what lies ahead. I was thirty-five years old, and up to that point, I had led a sheltered life. Most of my suffering had been existential, which meant I had to invent reasons to torture myself. Things generally came easily to me, just the way conception had. I awoke each morning believing in the inviolability of my identity, and of my rights.

In the hospital I am transferred smoothly from one nurse to another to another. They handle me as if I am a museum piece that they are responsible for moving, but one of only middling value. (This is somehow reassuring. My case is not important enough to be treated with special consideration.) I am hooked up to a machine with huge suction cups attached to my belly. The machine churns out a long scroll and blinks red numbers in its two eyes, my heartbeat and my baby's. To me, all machines possess a cruel, implacable air, even everyday ones like elevators and alarm clocks. But I have been hooked up to this one before; it is called an external fetal monitor. I remember the technician last week who told me my baby was "sluggish" and kept feeding me chocolate Kisses and making loud noises directed at my stomach with something that looked like a bullhorn. I hope, in a Winnie-the-Poohish sort of way, that someone will bring me chocolate Kisses now, but nobody does. Instead a midwife arrives and promptly sticks her fist up me. Some tarry, clotted stuff smears her rubber glove when she pulls out of me. "Look, bloody show," she says. The shock of my first blood silences me. She waits for my reaction— wanting to please, I search desperately through my store of etiquette. How, how does one find the right expression for bloody show?

While this is going on, my husband is eating from the plate of lunch they have brought in for us. He eats from my tray also, shoveling in the congealed mashed potatoes and fried chicken that I have only picked at. His hunger reveals a strong instinct for self-preservation, which I now find offensive. I turn away from the sight of him eating. Mountainous and soiled as I am, I am still a delicate creature.

The machine reveals, not surprisingly, that my baby is somewhat under stress. I will have to remain hooked up to the monitor "at least temporarily." I am alarmed, because my claustrophobia is flaring up. I feel sorry for my baby, who must be feeling even more closed in than I am. But I cannot afford to waste much energy on him right now. Suddenly he does not seem to be the point.

I am ushered into my labor and delivery room by a chubby nurse with red cheeks and buckteeth, who tells me to change into a gown. "Giving birth is very messy," she informs me. My curiosity is piqued (just how much messier can it get? how much farther will my dignity be compromised?). Just before I lie down, I glance out the window, with its gorgeous view of the Golden Gate Bridge and the Marin headlands and the fog curling up over the bay. It is the last time I will notice this view, that I so naively looked forward to enjoying. The nurses who pop in and out over the course of the next twenty hours make endless chit-chat—will the fog clear? had anybody ever seen such dismal weather so early in winter? do you think it's snowing in the mountains?—and I begin to think they are all insane.

The first machine is compounded by a second machine, and then a third. A hard-jawed M.D. decides she will have to break my water in order to keep the baby from being infected by his own feces. When the water is broken—a greenish-black oozing mass of swampish fluid, according to my husband, although I don't look—I am told that water will have to be put back *in* again, for reasons I cannot fully grasp, as my mind can only function clearly in the brief intervals between pain. The midwives and doctors wait politely for me to finish a contraction before continuing their explanations.

I am hooked up to a catheter, and an IV pumps fluids into my veins. Plastic bags with thin tubes hover over my body like aliens from outer space; they are neither benign nor hostile, simply watchful. "The pain is awful," I say to the midwife, who nods sympathetically, but without much interest. I know this is a foolish thing to say, but I can't help myself. Pain is the currency here, it is scattered everywhere like pennies, it has no special value. She casually suggests an epidural, but I recoil. That would mean failure! In my nine months of preparation for this moment, I had never imagined giving in to drugs. There is a certain *macha* status granted to women who give birth "naturally" and I want my badge. My cervix, however, is not cooperating.

I surrender by stubborn degrees. I accept one shot of Demerol and then another as I sit up in a chair (the tubes and wobbly bags follow me faithfully wherever I go). The Demerol does not take away the pain, exactly, but it makes me forget about it, at least while the shot lasts, and I feel queenly sitting there ordering my husband to bring me ice chips or to bathe my forehead. "This isn't so bad," I tell him and he nods grimly, washcloth in hand. Betty, the night nurse, coaches my breathing, which turns out to be all wrong. "Try to focus on your cervix opening, imagine it stretching with each breath, a little more and then a little more." I try, but my imagination is not up to the task—I am much more interested in a lollipop someone has given me to relieve my dry mouth. What is the cervix? Who has ever seen it? Does it really exist? Ice chips, my husband's broad warm hand, Betty's stern pug nose, the pungent sweetness of the candy—these are my realities at the moment. The lollipop dyes my lips and tongue a hideous blue that I am told lingers right up until I deliver.

I don't know if it's day or night. My days no longer have an end or middle or beginning, nothing I can grasp on to in order to orient myself (time to floss my teeth, time to eat a snack); they are simply one long, long minute repeating itself over and over again. Nothing is familiar, not even the hands of a clock.

"How are you doing?" asks my midwife.

"Wonderful," I pant. I grimace and show her my blue lips. "Give me another shot of Demerol, please."

"Now listen to me," she says, "I have to tell you something. We're going to have to give you Pitocin. It's a drug that speeds up your contractions. Your cervix is not dilating properly, and this will help. But you'll probably need the epidural."

An epidural blocks all feeling below the waist, makes you lose the use of your legs. Will I have to be paralyzed on top of everything else?

It is night by now—too dark for the nurses to discuss the weather. I have been in labor over twenty-four hours, and it is high time to submit. At some stage of extreme physical stress, you start to objectify yourself: your body is not yours anymore, but something that others are doing things to. It is better, in these situations, to offer yourself up as quickly as possible. All of the things that follow seem to be happening on a stage floating somewhere just to the side of or just below my body. I am both actor and critic, and in both roles I am somewhat detached.

Now I am introduced to the anesthesiologist, who travels from birthing room to birthing room like a visiting god. He is Vietnamese: slender, with honey-colored skin, a smooth-planed face, and beautifully molded hands. I immediately fall madly in love with him. Like the others, he speaks to me between contractions, waiting ever so calmly and politely.

"Sit up on the bed and remain very still," he instructs me in his lovely silky voice. "You must not move. I am going to insert a catheter into your spine through which the drug will flow. Hold onto your husband's hands; he will steady you."

He stands behind me and lifts my hospital gown. This gives me a small erotic thrill. My back feels naked and cool. My husband stands in front of me, and I bow and grip his hands. An odd configuration—the anesthesiologist behind me, poised with a needle, me in the middle, in the posture of a supplicant, my husband in front, bull-like and steady, my pain flowing into his strong forearms.

The relief is instantaneous. And it is swiftly followed by terror when I realize that my legs are becoming heavy and useless. The nurses and midwives lay me gently down on the table, disentangling all the different cords. A fourth machine joins the three already hovering over me with their watchful and what I now think of as slightly skeptical air. (Will this birth happen? Does this woman have sufficient moral fiber to bring new life into the world?) This one administers the contraction-inducing drug intravenously; the flashing red lights measure the strength of my contractions, which I now experience without feeling. If I choose, I can keep track of my progress on a screen—but as with the visualization of my cervix, I simply can't muster enough interest. Cheerfully a nurse tells me I will be able to sleep now; my womb will contract without my participation. I decide that unconsciousness is a viable option—I have already submitted this much, why not a little further? My husband amuses himself by announcing the strength of my contractions with the cheerful air of a sports announcer, but after awhile he curls up on the couch next to my bed and sleeps.

We are both jolted awake by the noise from the birthing room next door. "God help me! God help me!" screams a woman. A pattering of feet down the hallway, scuffling. The woman screams again. Suddenly I feel my own pains shooting down my back and thighs; the anesthesia is wearing off. "They're coming back!" I yell. I begin pressing all the buttons I can find. I struggle with my bonds, but I cannot escape. I am forced to hear the woman give birth: sobs, bone-chilling curses, and a final bloodcurdling howl. In all the chaos I forget to listen for the sound of an infant crying.

Some time before dawn I come down with a violent attack of chills. My thirst is hellish, bottomless; I beg my husband for glass after glass of water, and for blankets. A nurse pumps antibiotics into me—yet another IV!—and then administers Tylenol in suppository form, pushing it in briskly with her thumb. This night nurse is fat and blowzy—her gray frizzed hair, her scattered, incoherent words, and her unclean appearance make me uneasy. She is a bad omen.

By morning I am still only six centimeters dilated, not enough for the final push. Three doctors and two midwives stand in the hallway consulting, and I hear the word: "Caesarean." No more pretending that I can have a normal birth now. My obstetrician is Irish, with an enthusiastic expression, florid skin, and a refreshed air, as if she has just taken a dip in a cool mountain stream. She has been summoned from her warm bed in order to plunge her strong peasant's arms into my enormous belly. She looks quite capable of doing this, as well as quite sane. I make up my mind to let her have me.

Let them have me. My legs, my neurological system, my veins, my various orifices. Only the contents of my womb belong wholly to me—surely this must be true. Consent forms are propped up under my nose to sign. The anesthesiologist pumps more elixir into my spinal cord. This time the concentration of the drug is so powerful that I can no longer even wiggle my toes. I beg for a sedative.

I am wheeled into an operating room and rolled onto another table. Out of nowhere my husband appears in blue scrubs and gloves and a mask, his curly hair very spry, and I am struck by how handsome he is just then. His arms look meaty and confident, as if they know just what to do with my swollen belly. It occurs to me all of a sudden that I would like to sleep with him. But I can't, because I'm paralyzed from the waist down, and I am about to be sliced into. Morphine and a spinal block have confused me; why else would I become randy at such an inconvenient time? I mourn because I cannot have sex with my husband. I feel abandoned—or perhaps I am the one who is doing the abandoning, who knows?

A Caesarean does not take long; it is all the building up to it that is dramatic. It is anticlimactic in some ways. A screen is erected over my waist—I feel cut in half, like a magician's assistant—and about five thousand doctors gather at one end of me and five thousand at the other. All the familiar faces from the last thirty hours are here to witness the finale. My husband peers over the screen and takes photos of blood and yellow fatty tissue and a gray, thickly twisting umbilical cord. I try to rest as advised; it is all being taken care of without me. My role is to lie still. Fifteen minutes later I hear a baby crying.

I stir. What is this? Is it something connected with me, or is it, like everything else, carrying on without my participation? I strain, lift my head; the crying noise moves farther away. My husband appears at my side. "He's got curly hair," he says excitedly. "And he scored nine out of ten on his Apgar test. He's got *very* big feet." So there *is* a baby. Do I smile, do I weep? What's appropriate? I try to sort out my reactions, to make them fit, but it's hopeless, I'm too muddled by drugs. When they bring our son, bundled and howling, close to my shoulder so that I can finally see him, I do feel a distinct *thwang* of relief. He is *out*. I am *alive*. One hundred years ago in this country, one third of all births ended in the mother's death. Hemorrhage, exhaustion, heart failure, blood poisoning, infection. I ought to feel grateful to that woman now peeling off her soiled latex gloves and scrubbing up. (Whistling an Irish tune as she does so.) But instead of simple gratitude, I am visited by a strange presentiment: is this the beginning of a lifetime of dependency on doctors?

My life, my baby's life, were never in serious danger, thanks to modern medicine. But for the space of thirty hours or so my identity, the signals and signposts by which I have always recognized my own essential nature as separate from the nature of all other conscious beings, has been held hostage and subjected to a profound dismantling of its mechanism. It is returned to me, with all parts working, but like a grandfather clock that has been taken apart and put back together, it doesn't strike quite the same note. In all outward appearances, I am still myself, but I will never be myself again. My husband doesn't know this yet. My baby, who has known me from the inside out, will perhaps guess but won't care; my essential nature is not of urgent importance to him right now. He wants breast, and soon. I am all alone with my little offbeat tune, the slightly out-of-kilter sensibility. I hold my son; I wait for a reaction, any reaction. But my sense of alienation from myself has impaired my emotions.

I realize that there is a before and after in my life, a nitty-gritty now and then. The Caesarean itself, so bloody, violent, final, is an apt metaphor for the line I have crossed. I squeeze my eyes shut, try to will myself back into the day before yesterday, to the evening I am serving whitefish in lemon sauce to my friends, to the giddy dismay of my first contractions—there was something I forgot to do in that time, something I forgot to say, some act I neglected to perform. But it's too late. It is at this exact moment and not a moment before that I suddenly realize I am going to become a mother. Yet I don't know how to be a mother, in spite of all the reading I have been doing. I have no more reserves to call upon, I am exhausted, but people expect more from me—and I don't know how I can possibly meet their demands.

The Caesarean dealt the final blow to my innocence. I had taken a book with me into the birthing room, thinking that I might read between contractions. And I had packed a pair of slim black velvet shoes to wear home after the birth, wanting something pretty after all the months of ungainliness. Not knowing that my feet would be swollen to three times their normal size, that I would have to, instead, wear my husband's sneakers as I shuffled down the hospital corridor, clutching my newborn baby all lopsided against my chest. Sometimes, in the years to follow, I thought of the person I was when I packed those black velvet slippers and that book and I was racked with nostalgia—did I say goodbye to her properly? That endearing young woman, with her foolish notions? Vain, but good-hearted all the same. She was gone, simply got lost in the commotion, and yet she deserved a more attentive farewell.

It will be months before I feel anything when I pick up my son. Like a machine, I am dull and efficient, changing diapers, breastfeeding, rocking and burping. After my first disillusionment in the delivery room, I learn to expect nothing from myself except this expert efficiency. It is enough for the time being. I hope that my poor baby, driven as he is by sheer expediency, will not notice my lack of sensation.

When the love does come, it is authentic, searing. A mobile hanging over my son's crib comes loose and drops on his face; his screams bring me running from the living room, where I am dozing over the *New York Times*, which I delude myself into believing that I am reading every day, although I am barely able to get past the headlines. As I tear the cardboard zebras and pandas from his face, hoping he is not smothered, that his eye has not been put out, that his forehead has not been scarred, as I gather him into my arms, I realize that I do indeed adore him. He is mine; I am his. I become aware, with relief, that I am a mother now. I wasn't before. It is a process that began during the Caesarean and has been continuing ever since. I am being forged anew. Little by little, I reinvent myself.

Chapter Two

Prognosis Guarded

There used to be many stories to tell, but now I have only one. The drama of illness is always central, relegating everything else to the status of subplot, or so it seems. Sometimes, also, illness provides a natural climax to life, in which all the details are disparate, chaotic, inconclusive. The fog clears, and we see what it was all leading to at last. Everything falls into place. A serious illness is a master dramatist, setting the pace and tone, arranging all the scenes with the practiced hand of an artist.

I was thirty-six years old, had been married nearly four years and had a baby eleven months old, when, out of the wild blue sky, I was diagnosed with full-blown AIDS. Before my diagnosis I had been sick all summer long, first with a bad case of sinusitis I had picked up from my baby, then with an ear infection. A hacking cough lingered for months. Mysterious fevers came and went like distant cousins. The sinusitis lasted two weeks; every day my fever would mount to 102 and make a slow descent by early evening to a less giddy level of 99, after massive doses of Tylenol. I could feel noxious fluids moving ponderously through the hidden channels of my skull, especially around my ears—slouching, taking their sweet time with me. Two nights in a row I woke up with my pajamas thoroughly soaked with sweat. A doctor gave me some antibiotics and told me I would be feeling better in forty-eight hours. I hung on for the magical forty-eight hours but they passed, and then seventy-two, and then ninety-six and the evil fluids backed off but did not release their grip on me completely. And then the ear infection blocked off the entire right side of my head, creating a pressure so intense it made my teeth hurt.

During all this time I continued nursing my little boy just as I had always done. It was a pleasure we both knew was over but could not give up the habit of, and he didn't seem to mind his mama's feverish breasts. I was reassured by several pediatricians that the antibiotics and decongestants I had begun to swallow by the handful every day would not harm him. I wasn't entirely convinced of this and felt guilty but I still couldn't stop. Breast milk laced with Sudafed is still better than no breast milk at all, I reasoned.

But what was wrong with me? The sinusitis finally retreated, and my ear infection cleared up, but I coughed so hard I saw stars and I got no sleep at night. I had lost a considerable amount of weight. My hair was falling out. Strange headaches, of a breed I'd never experienced before, plagued me. They weren't painful, exactly, but they felt like someone was taking the heel of their hands and pressing relentlessly against the area between my temple and jaw. Sometimes the headache moved from one side to the other, sometimes it attacked both sides simultaneously. The constancy of this sensation spun me into a claustrophobic panic: it was as if walls were closing in on me. Every day, regardless of whether or not I'd had a good night's sleep, I experienced a bone-numbing fatigue. On our daily excursions to Golden Gate Park, I would wait until my baby napped, then I would flop down on a blanket next to his carriage and fall into a deep sleep; I would wake up an hour later rubbing my eyes and staring at the tree branches above my head, feeling worse than before. And then panic would un-spool me again, each day at more unruly lengths, until I be-came unraveled altogether, a lapful of tangled yarn. What the *hell* was wrong with me? Every morning I set my sights on good health, steeling myself: "Today I'll be better. I *have* to get better, I have an infant to look after, I have no busi-ness being sick, no time for it. So I'm going to get well and that's that." Such resolve had always worked in the past when I needed to recover from a flu or cold, but it didn't work this time. I began to lose faith in myself.

One day, wheeling the carriage down the block toward our apartment, I began to sob and I cried out loud to my baby, "I'm going to die, I'm not going to live to see you grow up."

Shortly after this I received my terrible diagnosis. At first, like everyone who is dealt this kind of news, I believed there had been an error, and I kept a firm hold on this belief for three days, until they told me that my little boy had antibodies. Then there was no more fantasizing that they had mixed up my name—a fairly common one—with someone else's in the lab, someone who happened to be ex-actly my age and race and weight and who also happened, by some miraculous coincidence, to have a male child ex-actly my son's age, who bore my son's name. There was no mistake.

I stopped nursing immediately, on my pediatrician's ad-vice. "There is a 25 percent chance your son is infected," she told me, and a fancy pediatric immunologist who ex-amined my baby the morning after my diagnosis con-firmed this but added that positive antibodies meant noth-ing in a child so young; antibodies were always passed to an infant through the placenta, and a more in-depth test was available that would look for the presence of actual virus in his bloodstream. It turned out that my Caesarean delivery, which I had always been ashamed of, feeling that I had merely had a baby pulled out of me instead of giving birth to one, had actually been a safeguard for my child. The virus nestled in the walls of the birth canal and a fetus who did not make this treacherous passage stood a much better chance.

Results of my son's test would take several weeks to obtain. My husband's antibody tests were negative—which meant that he had not given the virus to me—but this test result was also inconclusive. We learned that a person who had been recently infected could still have a negative result on a standard antibody test—the body sometimes took as long as several months to produce antibodies to the HIV virus. We would have to wait for the results of his viral load test as well.

My breasts ached and wept thin bluish liquid. It was only in the last year that they had acquired their exalted status. They had always been adolescent, understated, light as butterflies on my chest. They did not tread too heavily on my consciousness. But when I was pregnant and later nursing, I fell madly in love with my breasts; I would often catch myself in public hefting them with my hands. I'm sure there was a demented smile on my face as I felt myself up on buses and street corners. They swelled over my ribcage; the nipples hung lower, accommodating themselves to my baby's mouth. The flesh near the areolas turned purple with ecstasy.

And now I was jolted into the realization that what I fondly imagined had been nurturing my son for many months had in fact been endangering his life. My little boy took to formula with gusto; apart from a few playful nips here and there, he quit nursing without any regrets. But my breasts grew angry and stony from backed up milk. I cried at the sight of myself.

I was started on treatment: three different drugs, amounting to fourteen pills a day and a prophylactic antibiotic taken three times a week, all of which came with multi-paged instructions that resembled treatises. As a sort of bonus, the doctors threw in tranquilizers, antidepressants, and sleeping pills. The drugs had names that sounded like evil characters in a science fiction movie, and the drug that was the most powerful of all—and which I was admonished to treat with the utmost respect and fidelity, to pay it homage three times each day, year in and year out, on an exact schedule without fail—was like the antichrist himself imprisoned in a powder-filled gelatin capsule. Its fearsome name prickled my tongue. I was counseled to seek psychiatric help; I was "depressed," according to my physicians. They were damned right: I *was* depressed. I was given my "counts"—viral load and T-cell—so that I could better know myself, or at least be better informed. The counts were not good. Apparently there was a holocaust in my bloodstream.

Having AIDS forces you to think about who you are or who you were, sexually and otherwise. You provided all the introductions, virus to healthy host; there was no accident involved, although there may have been varying levels of unconsciousness and ignorance, willful or otherwise. It is not like cancer or multiple sclerosis, a genetic mishap. In the crudest and most undigested way of perceiving it, *you destroyed your own health*. Children, victims of rape or infected blood transfusions, partners who contract it in what they believed was a monogamous relationship—I imagine that their mental burden is easier, although maybe only by small degrees. The rest of us, whoever we are, have to come to terms with our culpability. We have dealt our immune systems—and perhaps those of our loved ones—an enormous blow. Unintentionally, but, nevertheless, by our own hand. Those were the first thoughts that came to mind during the weeks that I waited to hear about the outcome of my son's and my husband's blood tests.

Who was I? Obviously I was not a gay man, and I had also never been anything resembling a prostitute or a drug user. I had been faithful to my husband and he to me. When I labored to call forth an image of my pre-diagnosis self—and this was a search and rescue mission, since the illness had savagely mauled my identity—the primary hues were radiant youth and health. The emotional dark green of cypress trees against the bright blue of a San Francisco sky, or the flinch of winter sun on snow in Chicago. My husband and I had been serious hikers, and before I had known him I used to walk two and a half miles to work and back every day, even in freezing weather. I had never smoked and secretly despised people who did, although I pretended to more openness than I felt on principle; I rarely touched alcohol and was more frightened than contemptuous of people who abused it. I had been slim all my life without trying to be, and I was envied for this; aware that I was envied, I had developed what I was ashamed to admit was a small leverage over other women because of this quality, which I imagined that I tried to downplay, although in reality, of course, I did nothing of the sort. In my later twenties I made more of a conscious effort to struggle against vanity, but either I was not guilty enough, or my vanity was unscalable like some mountains are, and I gave up and lapsed into my old bad habits of thinking very well of myself indeed. Occasionally I triumphed over my narcissism and was able to focus on external things. I read thoroughly and vigorously. I flexed my mind with opera and plays and lots of travel and hard work and writing.

As a young single woman, I was pretty in a more conventional sense than I had been as a child and teenager, and I took advantage of this also: I always had plenty of dates and boyfriends. I had come of age in the seventies; I instructed myself that pleasure was my right, and that sex and its attendant joys could be innocent and inconsequential. This was one of the enormous lies that polluted the air everybody of my generation grew up breathing, and I can hardly blame myself.

I did not know anyone who was seriously ill. My mother and father were alive and well. My grandparents had died, but they had lived in other cities and I had not witnessed their deaths. I had only been to one funeral, that of a great uncle whom I had not been close to. On a flimsy excuse I had not gone to my co-worker's mother's funeral, although I liked my co-worker very much and felt sorry for her. I turned my head if I saw someone in a wheelchair or someone passed out on the street; I wanted to be the sort of person who helped in an emergency, but instead, I was the sort of person who panicked and bolted. I read about illness— breast cancer, AIDS—in the papers and shuddered and turned the page. One always reads about these things, I reminded myself. It doesn't mean anything. Because it's not true, no one's sick—the earth is stirringly beautiful, pulsing with goodness. Disease is some sort of a mistake, especially in America—it's like making a minor error in balancing your checkbook, something silly. I was lucky and knew it. I pitied people who were not as lucky as me, but what could I really do for them? I was powerless to change their luck. All I could do was to go on energetically enjoying my life.

I was struck by the delusions embedded in this compounded self-image. My doctors told me that I had most certainly been HIV positive for many years—ten or more— by the time I was diagnosed. Now that I had the advantage of hindsight, I could look back and see all the places where I had stumbled by accident upon the truth and had hastily shoved it out of the way again. I reviewed each one of them with scrupulous care, for I was young and remembered everything that had happened to me, and certainly every-thing that had happened of a physiological nature. None of the complaints had been serious, but all had been odd. I counted them off on my fingers, and also each excuse I had made for them, doing a sort of penance. There had been the morning I had woken up in the arms of my graduate-school boyfriend and immediately mounted him for a morning tumble; we both noticed a strange purplish rash on my left thigh. As we watched in horror, it spread within minutes over my entire body. We had been eating oysters the night before; I assumed the rash was related. My boyfriend rushed me to the emergency room, where they told me I was not sick enough for it to be an allergic reaction to oysters; it was some virus, they said. What virus? A shrug of the shoulders. Some virus; not serious. This was 1985. It would clear up in a few days. It did. My best friend and I referred to the rash for years as my "spots." Whenever invited to partake of oys-ters, I refused and cheerfully offered the story of my "spots" as an excuse and a good tale all in one. It had never been a question of oysters, that I knew, but it was an easy, color-between-the-lines explanation. Besides, laughing about the rash helped put it in its place; it was always nudging at my consciousness. I never ate oysters again.

And then there were the frequent bladder infections I began to suffer from during the same love affair: not seri-ous, but annoying—the burning urge to pee that was still not satisfied even after you had peed, like some torture de-vised in a female hell, the sleepless nights and the pain. I put this off to a small bladder and the unfortunate side effects of the sponge as a method of contraception. There were menstrual periods that were heavy, sudden, and ominous, like Midwestern storms. In the winter, clown-like patches of red on my cheeks and irritating flakes around my nose and eyebrows. Dryness, I concluded. Aging. Over the course of a few years the texture of my hair changed in a disturbing manner; it became brittle and thinner. Cheap shampoo—won't buy the drugstore brand anymore, I promised myself. Aging again. Too violent and impulsive with the blow dryer; must be gentler.

One afternoon in the spring of 1991, my regular physician, breathing heavily through his adenoids, dug his fingers in the soft flesh under my arms and said rather crossly, "You have some lumps here." I looked over his shoulder at the framed print advertising some long-gone Monet exhibit at the Art Institute and thought: right behind those lily pads it's waiting for me—*death*. I went back to work, locked myself in my office, and sobbed to my best friend on the phone: the word "cancer" left a metallic taste in my mouth, as if I'd been sucking on a coin. I had a lymph node biopsy and the weekend after, while I waited for the results, I felt exposed and delicate, like a hothouse plant that has been moved too soon. I sat for long periods staring at nothing in the beautiful pink and green marble foyer of the new main branch of the Chicago library, where, for some reason, I had gone to contemplate the alien concept of my mortality. I was unattached at the time and I remember working myself into a state of tremendous pity for the suffering of my parents, who might have to outlive me. In a fit of nobility I decided to leave my money market account (ten thousand dollars inherited from my grandfather) and several IRAs to my dear friend, who came from a large family and would stand to inherit no money of her own. She could use the money as a down payment for a condo; she would never forget me, because I had been the one who had set her on the path of financial security. These two thoughts were the extent of my musing over death those afternoons in the brand-new, empty foyer of the public library.

The lymph nodes were benign. I asked briefly, "What are they then?" and was told, "Some infection, not important," but I did not pursue it further: the fact that it was not cancer was enough for me. I felt light and flexible once more, a bamboo pole, not a frail orchid. What joy! I was myself again—not a sick person after all! For the lymph nodes I made no excuse; I simply turned my back on them. Good health sprang into my arms and I welcomed it with revels. For years I did not give another thought to death.

But there were stomach complaints, some minor, some more serious. An increasing problem with indigestion and heartburn; once an episode of stabbing pain in the upper abdomen that a physician quickly diagnosed as an ulcer and that cleared up after a week of Maalox. A bad case of diarrhea when I was four months pregnant that finally drove me to take antibiotics.

And I could not forget the frightening case of shingles I'd had in 1993. A hot summer day and a backache, not untypical for me, but the backache metamorphosed into a tingling from my shoulder to mid-spine and the tingling erupted into an ugly diagonal row of raised red bumps. The pain was singeing. The internist on duty flashed me a wary, close-faced glance. All was not well. "Chicken pox virus," he said briefly. "But I've had the chicken pox, a long time ago," I replied. He shrugged. "Happens sometimes when the immune system is suppressed. Old people sometimes get it." He shrugged his shoulders. "Just happens sometimes." I spent a painful weekend with my husband in the Gold Country trying to forget about the nasty crusting sores on my back and, worse, the burning that left me twisting and turning constantly, seeking comfort. Industriously I suppressed the idea of the suppressed immune system—it just could not be. I'm married and I'm *very* healthy, I told myself. I hike and bike and take aerobics three times a week. I even floss my teeth twice a day. I'd caught something from the bums I brushed shoulders with on Muni or in Union Square. That was the explanation. I experienced a few moments of violent hatred for the homeless, for their relentless odors and urine-soaked rags and the invisible microbes they had passed along to me. When I got over the shingles I forgave them and for a month or so made a point of giving every homeless person I saw a pocketful of loose change.

Reviewing all this, I was stunned. All the while I had been identifying myself as a superlatively healthy young person, I had in reality been stalked by disease. By the age of twenty-five I was already a marked woman. All my confidence disappeared in shreds. Was it possible that the somewhat arrogant, thoughtful, innocently happy, intelligent and fleet-footed girl I had identified with was not me at all? My heart was broken. Instead of belonging to the world of the well, I belonged to the world of the sick. All these years had been mere playacting.

And because of this reckless self-confidence, my beloved child's life might be endangered. Yet it was because of this reckless self-confidence that he had been *born;* if I had known I was not healthy at the core, I would never have chosen to conceive. His sunburst smiles would be quenched by pain and illness; his plump delicious limbs would wither away. In the corridors of the clinic where I went to have round after round of tests, I saw a bald girl in a plaid dress huddled next to her mother, a plastic tube going up her nose. Had I brought a child into the world only for it to suffer? Suddenly it occurred to me that if AIDS could happen, then any disaster could. I saw my husband falling sick and losing his job, my parents killed in a car accident, my family being evicted from our apartment, my insurance bottoming out and the company refusing to pay for my treatments. We would go on welfare. I would beg. I re-read the story of Job and, weeping, saw myself in the tale of that unjustly punished man. Would I be able to follow Job's example of unparalleled faith? No, of course not. The worst punishment of all was the shattering of the faith I'd had in my ironclad youth.

I took to my bed, as they say in Victorian novels. I lay down and imagined what it would be like never to be able to get up again, not to be able to wash or feed myself or go to the bathroom. My parents and friends and my husband looked after my little boy while I went into deep mourning. I spent hours scrutinizing my body more obsessively than I ever had in the past, when the worst thing I was looking for was love handles. I spun into a panic over a bruise on my thumb and a freckle on my wrist. Each day when I woke up I groaned, thinking of the many long hours I would have to get through before I could go to sleep again. I suffered side effects from the medications and the pity I felt for myself for enduring them made me suffer from them more.

Feeling too Job-like, I visited the rabbi at a local synagogue. "What does suffering mean?" I asked her and she replied, after a moment's pause, "Suffering is what you make it." A little later I asked her, "But what should I do?" and she answered, "Spend as much time with your child as you can, without hovering over him." I was dissatisfied with these answers. I spotted a psychology text on her bookshelves: I had been looking for spiritual guidance, but a rabbi was nothing more than a cultured therapist after all. Later, after more reflection, I saw that she had given me the soundest advice that Judaism—or any religion—has to offer. But at the time I thought to myself, "She didn't even say she'd pray for me or my boy."

The mother of a close friend of mine sent me the history of Sister Bernadette and a small jar of holy water from Lourdes. This woman, in her late fifties, was contemplating joining a convent. The holy water made me laugh for the first time in months—so I suppose it really was holy. I tossed it on a pile of papers, to all appearances casually, but not really casually: I always knew exactly where it was, and was careful not to let it become buried under other things. Every now and then I checked on it, to make sure it was still there.

Slowly, I gained some ground. I tested negative for all of the serious opportunistic infections, including tuberculosis and PCP, and my doctor told me that I should consider myself lucky. In addition, I had become symptomatic during a period of frenetic research activity; the evil-sounding pill I swallowed on a strict schedule was considered nothing short of miraculous by the medical establishment, and even more brilliant drugs shimmered on the horizon.

I told myself I had the advantage of having contracted a very public and political disease that instantly conferred martyrdom upon its sufferers, whether they had earned it or not: for someone whose emotional life teetered on the brink of dramatics anyhow, the temptation to view myself on a par with, let's say, St. Francis of Assisi, was almost irresistible. What's more, this particular martyrdom was, paradoxically, a sociable kind. You could not have a more fashionable disease. In San Francisco, at least, the stigma was not as pronounced. Your civil rights were indisputable. Banners were raised in your honor; quilts were sewn; marathons were run; politicians' careers were made and broken; scientists trampled each other in the rush to the finish line. It was a crowded, noisy, up-to-the-minute kind of illness. Nearly thirty-four million people worldwide suffered from it.

But I was still all alone. It was not "my" disease. My whole life I had felt like I stood slightly askew of the mainstream, that I did not fully belong to any group that I had joined, and this was no different. I did not know anybody else like myself—white, Jewish, middle-class, college educated, and HIV positive. I tried turning it all upside down and thinking about it a different way. This was a more successful tactic. It was funny, but I had turned out to be exotic after all, just as I had secretly wanted to be. Wearing dirty sweat pants I flopped down on the couch, nauseated and exhausted, with a skull-piercing headache, listening to my little boy, who was just learning how to walk, patter up and down the hallway, and I thought to myself: I am so *distinguished*.

A single moment in time—perhaps shared with my graduate-school lover, perhaps with someone more insignificant—had awarded me this distinction. I wondered if I had been promiscuous. But then, what was promiscuous? I worried this point like a dog with an old bone and finally, like the dog, I buried it. Everybody must. Promiscuity is a relative term that in the end proves useless. I did not know who had given me the disease, but I discovered, to my surprise, that I harbored no revenge fantasies about this man, whoever he was. In any case, I was certain that whoever had infected me had not known that he was infected himself, and so he was in the same boat I was, if he were still alive. I was willing to take full responsibility for my illness: that seemed the least I could do to appease the gods. I had always been an introspective person; *I'll get to the bottom of this,* I promised. Job too had asked himself the universal question—why me?—and, finding no answer, had concluded *just because it is so*—but I was not satisfied with that. There had to be an explanation.

I could not read more than a paragraph at a time or talk

to someone for ten minutes on the phone without my mind wandering; my head was splitting; I could not even concentrate on a half-hour cotton candy show on T.V. I was afraid I was going mad.

Then one day I was called to the phone: I knew immediately that it was my son's doctor. "Move your arms and legs now," I told myself, "walk," and I did not so much walk as maneuver myself toward the receiver, as if I were making my way through the alien atmosphere of another galaxy. "I have the results of your son's test," my pediatrician told me in her gentle, slightly lisping voice. I began to sob into the phone. Suddenly, with a relentless plummet, I was back in gravity's hold again. "He shows no trace of the virus," she said. I pressed the phone against my jaw and sobbed with more force. The pediatrician quickly said goodbye and hung up. I fondled the receiver a few more moments before letting it go. Then I immediately called my husband, who told me that he too had been informed that his blood showed no trace of the virus.

After this news, my health improved daily. I did not understand this deliverance any more than I understood why I had been forced to undergo such purgatory in the first place, but one thing I did know: I did not have the stamina to unravel the mystery. Not at that point, anyhow. My mind was not sufficiently evolved; I was no Jewish sage or Buddhist priest. I gave up the search for an explanation and concluded that Job, also, might simply have chosen resignation to his fate out of exhaustion—after all, what he'd undergone had sapped his physical strength and mental acuity. When I did think about what my faultline may have been, I concluded that it had been mostly naïveté—having lived a rather sheltered existence, I assumed that the world was a benign place, when actually it wasn't. And many of my sexual adventures had been prompted by a need to prove something about myself, although what it was I was trying to prove I could no longer remember. My life had gotten away from me at times; I had veered off track, and I assumed that in some vague cosmic way I was being punished for this. This was the outer limit of my philosophizing.

I gained weight; food tasted like food again instead of sawdust; my headaches disappeared. I concentrated on gratitude. Everyday life, with all its delicious pleasures, resumed. I took my rabbi's advice and returned to my child both emotionally and physically. One thing I did gain, which I could point to: I had no more ambivalent feelings about motherhood. There was nothing common or animal-like about it. Giving birth had not been a sacrifice of my higher nature, as I had once half-believed, but a redemption of that higher nature and an enhancement of it. Particularly in my case, the birth of a healthy child was nothing to take for granted. I was more of a person, not less. Other women had known this for thousands of years; but I had always been stubborn and would never take anybody's word for anything. It was liberating to be so free of doubt, to know exactly where I stood. I rejoiced.

My doctor wrote on the disability form I asked her to fill out, "Prognosis guarded." That single adjective made me weep bitterly. I mailed the form off quickly so as not to have to look at it anymore—safe in the hands of the U.S. Postal Service, perhaps its message would lose its potency. But it was too late: I had taken the words to heart. From then on I would always be a person who was guarded, both by doctors and myself. I held myself carefully positioned toward life: the angle had to be just so. No more carefree poses. I kept a wary eye on the opposite party; that was all I could do.

Chapter Three

Doctors I Have Known

Well, to begin, there was the doctor who diagnosed me with tuberculosis when I was five years old. I don't remember him, although I have an impression of him being haughty and portly and wearing a vest with a watch chain. This image may have been superimposed upon my memory later, however, as the result of having read too many Victorian novels. He had the reputation of being a prince among pediatricians, according to a friend of my mother's. Sometimes he drew me pictures of bunnies or ducks, which seems a fantastic thing for a doctor to do. I understand he also made house calls, but I don't remember any of these.

I did not suffer at all from the tuberculosis; luckily, treatment was available. But for many months after the treatment was completed, I had to visit the hospital regularly for a sputum check. The procedure involved forcing tubes down my nostrils and since I was a small child they wanted to strap me on a table. I don't remember any of the doctors who attempted to hold me down but I remember doing wild battle against them. I retain an image of a harried woman with stringy black hair who argued with my mother that the strapping was absolutely necessary. My mother insisted that *nobody* was going to strap me down and that I would stay still all by myself, if only they would stop trying to force me into bondage. She won; they didn't strap me down, and I did stay still. After it was over I wept bitterly in my father's arms and was given Bazooka bubble gum as a bravery reward.

My first pediatrician retired and I went to another pediatrician whom I saw until I was seventeen years old and went away to college. He was comical, sharp-witted, Jewish, and he knew just how to handle my mother, who attended me in the examining room until I was fourteen and I finally rebelled and insisted on going solo. He told jokes; I have no memory of any other doctor, before or since, telling jokes. Doctoring became a grimmer business, apparently, somewhere during the mid-seventies. The nurse who sat behind the glass booth in the reception area and who assisted him in various procedures was rumored to be his wife, although no trace of this relationship could be detected within the office. They addressed each other as "Doctor" and "Nurse." She was tall and straight-backed and supremely neat. She was wry to his effusive funniness; they were a satisfying match. She wore a white uniform and, of all things, a cap.

This doctor had a waiting room with colored plastic chairs and a table stacked with shabby copies of *Highlights* and *Jack and Jill*. If you wanted to go to the bathroom, the nurse handed you a key on a long wooden paddle and sent you down a hallway that smelled of mildew. This reception area was where I first perfected the art of waiting for doctors. The wait was never long. Soon the door to the inner offices would open and you would be summoned. I never waited in the actual examining room the way I did many years later in large clinics, where one had to suffer waiting not once, but twice—in the Outer Office and again Within. Double waiting seemed to be a side effect of the exponential leaps medicine had taken during my young womanhood: they knew so much more, but as a result they were busier, so somebody who was somehow *not* your physician took your blood pressure and your temperature and then left you hanging.

I was never seriously ill again as a child or a teenager, although after the tuberculosis I developed the reputation of being delicate. I cultivated this reputation carefully for its romantic value; my actual health was robust. My funny pediatrician joked away all my complaints. He vaccinated me, saw me through chicken pox, influenza, colds, and other assorted viruses, and sent me on my way. Whatever became of him? I hope that he is alive and as jovial as ever and residing somewhere happily with his straight-backed nurse/wife.

There was a long hazy period during college and later graduate school when I had no doctor at all. Instead, I went to Student Health. Student Health was a precursor of Health Maintenance Organizations, which turned out to be my future. The clinics at Brandeis University and at the University of Michigan in Ann Arbor were where I first encountered interns, residents, medical students who "looked in" on your exam, and nurse practitioners. I don't remember a single one of these people, not one face. Of course, my health was always excellent, in spite of terrible eating and sleeping habits and the sexual and domestic chaos of dormitories, where young people of both genders were packed in dozens of tiny rooms in enormous ugly structures like gargantuan rabbit warrens. To think of my immune system, and all it withstood! I am envious, looking back: I took it so much for granted. I was fitted for a diaphragm, peed in a bottle for several pregnancy tests (false alarms), was handed codeine for a bad cough once or twice. That was my experience of Student Health. For many years I was never sick.

I did used to have terrible problems with impacted wax

in my ears, because my ear canals were unusually narrow, making drainage difficult. At least once a year I was driven to visit an otolaryngologist when general practitioners were unable to relieve me by the standard procedure of washing out my ears with a giant syringe. I was referred to one for an especially bad episode when I was living in Chicago in the years between college and graduate school. The ear man had a swank office on Michigan Avenue with chrome fixtures and miles of spotless gray carpeting. I was twenty-four years old. When he introduced himself, he said, "I don't really do this kind of thing anymore, I'm developing a practice in plastic surgery. But since you were referred, I'll examine you." He searched my face. "You're such an attractive young woman and you're walking around with acne scarring on your jaw—I could help you with that." I began to cry. My ear hurt.

He said, "What are you crying for?"

"You made me feel bad," I answered.

His mouth twisted with disgust. In silence he examined my ear. He was a bald, bulging-eyed little man—exactly the way he deserved to look, I thought.

"You have a severe infection," he said with some urgency and he summoned his assistant, an impossibly beautiful woman whose blondeness shone so hard I couldn't look at her. While he fished white pus out of my ear she stood by and held a receptacle.

He deigned to see me for a follow-up visit in a week. This time I was ready for him. He said to me, "Your ear is fine now. Have you thought anymore about cosmetic surgery?"

I answered, "I've had those scars since I was fourteen years old and I can live with them, thanks."

Again the wry twist of the mouth. He was finished with me in every sense—medical, commercial, human—but he patted my behind as I walked out of his office. If it had been the 1990s I could have made my fortune. But it was only 1984, and sexual harassment hadn't been invented yet.

My discussion of ear wax would not be complete without mentioning a general practitioner I visited in the small town of Grindelwald in Switzerland. My husband and I had just arrived from Zurich; we were on the first day of our honeymoon, dragged out with jet lag, and my right ear had been blocked and painful during the long flight overseas. I thought our vacation would be spoiled. While my husband slept in our lodgings I trudged up a steep hill to the clinic. On my left was the magnificent Eiger. The office was bright with yellow Swiss sunlight and empty; I was momentarily frightened. The doctor saw me right away: another bad sign. He looked like an aging Nazi, someone who might have favored eugenics—thinning blond hair, fleshed-out body—and his accent terrified me. A fitting end for a nice Jewish girl from America. I trembled. "Agh, what's the trouble, you're not a baby," he said. "Remain still, if you please." In two minutes he cleared up my problem. Instead of a Nazi he began to look to me more like tight-assed, tight-buttoned Christopher Plummer from *The Sound of Music*. "Go, go hike now," he said, waving his hand at the window and turning his back on me.

My unstuffed ears rang with newness and clarity. Perhaps it was the efficacy of the resolution that satisfied me so much; doctors at that moment seemed to be the best that they could be. Diagnosis and then, in the space of a few moments, cure—I grasped, in a flash, the beauty of the medical profession. The ideal of the cure, which seems so remote to me now, was so immediate then it was palpable.

And, some years later, there was the friendly ear specialist in San Francisco who amused my nine-month old baby with Yiddish nonsense words. I was the one who was sick, but he tolerated the presence of my child because I had no baby-sitter. He was patient with me—I had been running to him all summer long, desperate, and he kept reassuring me that nothing was wrong. "You're on the road to recovery," he said, slapping his hands on his legs. His confidence inspired me. I almost believed him. Of course, he had no idea what was really wrong with me.

In my mid-twenties I finally settled down with one doctor after a long period of flitting from one to the other, and this medical monogamy on my part was as comfortable and productive as the monogamy I later discovered in marriage. I belonged to an HMO in Chicago; since I was in perfect health and therefore not very fussy about doctors (I'd only be seeing them once a year or so, I figured), I called the patient representative and had her choose a primary care physician for me. It was a bit like matchmaking.

The doctor who had been arranged for me was close to my age, a tall man with a shuffling gait and a lantern jaw. I would hear his large feet slapping on the floor outside the corridor before he entered the examining room. His face was battle-scarred with acne; his simian arms were covered with black hair. He was one of the ugliest human beings I had ever seen, but as the years went on his ugliness began to seem strangely appealing. He lacked even a scrap of bedside manner, but this too aroused my sympathy and I decided to trust him. I stuck by him. I imagined him during his acne-bound years burying himself in his books and deciding he would go to medical school and tell everybody who had made fun of him to go fuck themselves.

It was around this time that I began to wonder more about doctors—where they lived, what they ate, what they read and dreamed about. And I began to wonder how they saw me, not as a patient (I already knew that), but as a human being. The barrier between my humanity and the doctor's humanity was profound. There it stood between us, invisible, on the office desk, although we could see the pores on each other's noses, were close enough to touch— and of course I *was* touched, many times. They had a *license* that proved they could touch me, but I was somehow not licensed to touch back.

What did I reveal about myself to my doctor in Chicago? More than he revealed about himself, certainly, and yet in many ways nothing at all. I visited him religiously once a year for a complete physical work-up. This included a gynecological exam, during which he palpated my breasts and took a Pap smear. In those days I always went to male gynecologists and thought nothing of it. A few years after I became his patient he informed me that a nurse would be attending during this portion of the exam, which must have meant there was something nasty in the air, something hurtful to us all. And after I moved to San Francisco in the early 1990s I was never given a gynecological exam by a man again.

My Chicago doctor asked me the same questions year after year. "Are you sexually active?"

"Yes," I'd say with casual pride. (I always wondered if *he* was.)

He asked me about my periods and birth control. He only mentioned condoms to me when I began to get frequent bladder infections. He asked me if the infections were the result of "intercourse" and when I answered yes he said to me grimly, "You should use condoms." He never explained why, although I understood the concept. He never spoke of AIDS to me; not a medical soul in Chicago ever did.

He addressed me as "Ms. Peterson," as in "What can I do for you today, Ms. Peterson?" when he answered my telephone calls—a responsibility that he always took upon himself, by the way, without passing my calls along to an advice nurse. I enjoyed this quaint formality. When I moved to San Francisco all doctors called me by my first name as if we'd just struck up a jolly acquaintance, yet at the same time there were far more rules and regulations for us both to abide by.

It was this doctor who first discovered, during a routine physical, the swollen lymph nodes under my armpits.

"It's the result of some kind of infection," he said.

"What kind of infection?" I asked him.

He didn't know. He asked me if I worked with children, if I had recently had a cut on my arm.

"It's fairly common, nothing to worry about really," he said.

He told me to keep an eye on it for a few weeks, but I could not live through that few weeks, and I called him from work one day and said, "I can't stop thinking about them."

"You're really freaking out about this, aren't you?" he said. I was touched by his use of the term "freaking out." It seemed a major step forward in the terms of our relationship; his allowing himself to embrace this slang term was an indication of his growing ease with me, a friendliness that had not been there in the past.

Eventually he referred me to a surgeon who did a biopsy. It was my first experience with surgeons and surgery. This man was too handsome: reddish hair, young and muscular. The lymph nodes turned out to be benign, but I went to the surgeon for one more visit to make sure the incision under my arm was healing properly. I was naked from the waist up and wore a hospital gown tied at the side; he walked into the room and observed me for a moment, then approached.

"The gown," he said, lowering his eyes.

I tried to untie it but I fumbled; he reached down himself and his fingers joined mine and together we undid the strings, impatiently. The gown fell around my waist.

"Put your hands on my shoulders," he instructed me. He moved very close. I did as he said. I let my arms go limp; I looked carefully around his head, although I wanted badly to look into his eyes. My mouth was an inch away from the lobe of his ear. He examined me.

He was deft, a good surgeon. "You're fine, doing well," he said and sprang to the other side of the room, putting his hands behind his back.

Had he taken a liberty with me, amused himself a bit? I don't know. He had both touched me and not touched me, that was what made the whole experience so sexy.

I did manage to compose myself enough to ask him if he knew why my lymph nodes had been acting up and he shrugged his shoulders and said, "It happens sometimes." This was an anticlimactic end to all the commotion of the operating room, but it satisfied me and for the time being I forgot all about them.

During this era I dated several doctors, and they were all odd fellows. One had survived the rigors of medical school and internship and had suddenly decided that he didn't like being a doctor and would rather have been a lawyer instead. He was an Orthodox Jew into the bargain; these contradictions in his character—the adherence to a very difficult form of Judaism and a flippancy toward his years of studies—troubled me and I soon stopped seeing him. Another had a chip on his shoulder because he'd been educated in Mexico. A third I was fixed up with while he was visiting relatives in Chicago; he was a budding neurologist, exact and polite. He took me to fine restaurants, made all the right sorts of dating conversation, gave me a peck on the cheek when he dropped me off. I was relieved when he went back to Toronto. We communicated for awhile but I didn't keep up my end of things sufficiently. I was informed by sources in the know that he became a great success and I might have married him. When I tried to imagine marriage to this man I pictured myself standing in a kitchen with a vast white tile floor and cabinets refurbished in maple and every appliance you could possibly dream up sparkling on the prodigious counters. I was glad I had not answered his last letter. Still, I was haunted occasionally by this doctor I didn't marry. What would my life have been like?

I never actually slept with a doctor. This is too bad, because it might have resolved some of my curiosity about them as human beings.

I had an acquaintance who was in medical school and he told me that doctors were no big deal and to get that myth out of my head once and for all. It was all a matter of memorization and discipline. They're just like you and me, he said. Modern science was the great thing; doctors were merely acolytes. At times in my life I believed him more than at other times.

Meanwhile I watched my homely doctor in Chicago gain in confidence. A wedding ring appeared on his left hand. By the time I myself married and moved to San Francisco, he was standing up straighter, did not bump into objects as he walked into the office, and seldom blushed when he asked me questions. He had blossomed professionally. Although he never guessed the real truth about me, it had been a mutually satisfying relationship. I forgive him for his ignorance, or his timidity. My general health was fine. His timidity may actually have been officially condoned by the medical establishment, so he wasn't to blame.

* * *

A few years later, in San Francisco, I had a doctor who said to me, "I know you, Paula." I wondered what exactly he meant by that. He knew my terrible diagnosis, but that wasn't it. Was he referring to my educational background, my personality, my instincts? My philosophy of life and illness, my sense of judgment? If so, how did he know these things, what had I said to reveal myself? He implied that he had recognized me somehow and I found this flattering. His remark probably had a far more limited explanation than I was imagining, but I liked him for it. One longs desperately all one's life to be known through and through.

There really was a doctor who did know me, or who at least observed me well. It happened only once. This was shortly after I had moved to San Francisco. He was a birdlike man who cocked his head when he spoke. He had given me a routine physical and he said to me, "You've got swollen lymph nodes everywhere, neck, groin, armpits. Ever been tested for HIV?"

I recoiled as if slapped. Shook my head.

"Are you an IV drug user? Ever had relations with a bisexual man?" He thrust his torso forward with a slightly defiant air, as if he sensed that his questions were unorthodox, an act of medical daring.

No. No, I replied.

"Night sweats? Fevers? Diarrhea?"

No. No. No.

"I'm *married*," I told him. I had found that doctors were often relieved when I told them this. They dropped the grim cautionary mask they had donned in my single days. They became more chatty.

He nodded politely. I had forgotten that I had already informed him of my marital status at the beginning of our conversation.

"Well, you might want to be tested, just to rule it out."

I refused, too fearful and unwilling to put myself through an agonizing emotional experience for what I imagined was little cause. He shrugged his shoulders and did not press the issue. He had done all he could do.

For a few minutes I had been in the presence of true medical astuteness. It was what I had always looked for from a doctor, but I did not appreciate it while it was happening to me. Such is life. I soon stopped seeing this man when I switched insurance plans.

My acquaintance with doctors accelerated in the next few years. I got pregnant and was introduced to a merry crew of midwives and nurse practitioners and the occasional female obstetrician whom I saw every several weeks for prenatal care. I performed for them all, peeing in cups, lumbering onto scales, thrusting out my arms and veins to have my blood drawn or pressure taken, climbing onto tables and obediently allowing myself to be hooked up to ultrasound machines and other ungainly medical instruments. During my labor and subsequent delivery by Caesarean section, all these jolly ladies seemed to whirl around me as if I were a giant Maypole; I remember being embarrassed by my immobility in the face of all this frantic activity. Finally, on my last day in the hospital, while I lay flat on my back, a man materialized at my bedside. He was the first male doctor I had seen in the maternity ward. He was tall and much older than everybody else and had an Olympian air of invulnerability.

"Are you ready to go home?" he asked me.

I didn't see how I could, but I nodded. He seemed to demand obedience.

"Well, we'll discharge you, then." He leaned a little

closer. "But just remember—save your energy, because taking care of a baby is a twenty-four-hour-a-day job."

I whispered, "Yes."

He seemed satisfied. He disappeared as mysteriously as he had arrived and I never saw him again, anywhere. He had gone back to Olympus. Did he actually still deliver babies, I wondered, or just preside over women who recently had? I imagined there was some secret wisdom he had been trying to impart to me, and I strained to catch hold of it.

There was my new "steady" physician, someone I had chosen because his name sounded comfortably Jewish and familiar, and because he had earned a degree in medicine, as opposed to nurse practitioners, who knew as much (I came to realize) but did not look as good on paper. He was young, the way they all were at the teaching hospital I had hooked up with, and his handsome, symmetrical features vaguely resembled those of a movie star who was currently in vogue. On the other hand he was not stunning enough to be bothersome, like the surgeon, and his manner was composed more of modest confidence than arrogance. His sufficient good looks and charm were a relief after my years with the Chicago practitioner: I did not think I had the patience to break in yet another doctor. I knew within thirty seconds of meeting him that I liked him: I had learned to trust my instincts with doctors. We chatted about my pregnancy, his two children, my job, my nagging stomach troubles, my general health. It was all very pleasant. He was conversationally talented. I liked passing time with him and I remember thinking that I would like to have a real talk with him, one not limited to my health. I imagined bumping into him, between the stacks in the medical library, or in front of the counter in the campus deli, and having a lively, spirited discussion about some subject of mutual interest.

It was this doctor who, a year and a half later, on an

unusually hot day in October, gave me my diagnosis. I was very thin and wore a white dress that, over the last several months, had become several sizes too large. I was a novitiate receiving her orders. "I have harsh news for you," he said, closing the door behind him after a brief mysterious absence from the examining room. I remember the writerly side of me appreciated the sensitivity that had gone into the word choice of "harsh" rather than "bad" or "upsetting." It was almost literary, and it confirmed my already good opinion of him. The other me rocked and hugged my shoulders and for some reason quite disturbing invoked the name of Christ. He watched me. The flesh beneath his eyes swelled with incipient tears. I loved him for that.

Unfortunately I had not had access to him all summer when I was feeling so ill. He was training medical students in Japan, and when he returned he took a vacation with his family. In the meantime I visited doctors on call, residents, screening clinic professionals. My chest was x-rayed, my blood was drawn and redrawn yet again. CT scans were taken of my head. Nothing of any significance was found to be wrong with me and a young pretty resident with a downy upper lip asked me politely if I might be suffering from depression. I could tell someone had been coaching her, or that she had been doing a lot of homework.

I had always thought of myself as an articulate person. But now I began to doubt myself. Something, obviously, had gone awry in my body: had something also gone awry with the channels of communication? There was the long-haired, jaded doctor in the emergency clinic who condescended to inform me, the night after I had bad chills which progressed to a fever of 103, that mothers of young children were always getting sick, and suggested that there might be some environmental factor behind my persistent cough, such as dust in my hallways. "You took your temperature?"

he said in disbelief. "I was freezing cold, I couldn't get warm with five blankets on me, I knew there was something wrong," I told him. He shrugged his shoulders. There was a vicious Filipino nurse who scowled when I stumbled into the clinic for the umpteenth time and wept, begging her to let me see a doctor, any doctor, right away.

Perhaps the fault was on my end. I labored harder to explain myself. I sat up nights revising my story for my next visit to the clinic, adjusting the angle, adding new details, in the desperate hope that by altering the form of my tale somewhat the essence might be better grasped. I was sick. That seemed so clear. And so it must have been language that was my stumbling block. A black gay male nurse rolled his eyes when I told him about my headaches and said, "You have chronic sinusitis." I told him the CT scan showed this wasn't so. He giggled and said, "I guess they're right then."

I tried pretending there was nothing wrong with me, that I was just a stressed-out, neurotic new mother who needed Xanax, not antibiotics. This tactic provided some faint comfort for a few days—although I did not much like the image of myself as a woman having a nervous breakdown, it was better than some other alternatives—but my confidence in my mental illness soon dwindled the next time a fever ravaged my body like a stormtrooper. If I was crazy, couldn't I be crazy without feeling so lousy, for God's sake? I abandoned this approach.

When my good doctor finally told me I had AIDS, I pointed to my head and said, "So this is not all psychological?"

"You had an intuition," he said, with his serious, sad expression.

Finally, my intuitions had been legitimized by the medical institution. I took strange pride in proving that I had been right all along. Then, almost immediately, after months of having been a low-level problem to the clinic, I became the center of attention. I found myself seated in an examining room with my husband next to me, my child in diapers on my knee, and in front of us, arranged in a polite semicircle at some distance, as if assembled for a chamber music performance, a small troupe of doctors, social workers, nurses and nurse practitioners. In the center was a South American Jewish pediatrician with a sexy accent but a disappointing pockmarked face. You could fall in love with him, but only over the phone. He told me that my baby was almost certainly fine, but me—me, ah, that was another question. He implied that from now on, I would never be able to do without doctors in my life. Much later, when I was able to reflect on the experience, I wondered how this new crew saw me—wondered how I was as an act, so to speak. Ordinary, I figured. They had seen this show before. Baby on the knee, buoyant and innocent of anticipatory fear, the stricken mother, the blunt and dismayed father. I knew all my lines and they, too, knew all their responses by heart. Still, they were kind. In some important way, I felt, their intelligent and informed sympathy would see me through. Their sympathy was no less genuine because it was professional and repeated on a daily basis.

Out of this haze of new faces a particular one materialized. She was the nurse practitioner to whom I had been assigned at the special clinic to which I had been handed over. At first I was blinded by fear, but after awhile my eyes cleared and there she was, sitting in a chair diagonally across from me, watching me with a keen, guarded glance (that expression so specific to medical folk), slender hands in her lap. She was attractive and slim and quick; her eyes were green-blue, her manner direct and incisive, and she had a stern compassion that steadied me even as it shook me from head to toe. She was sometimes rushed and forgot to hide this from me, and I felt like Alice in Wonderland who, in the first leg of her journey, meets the White Rabbit who runs by muttering, "No time to lose, no time to lose." But she had been on the front lines. Her sense of irony was well developed. Her sharp eyes scanned me, reading for meaning in every inch of my flesh—the flaky skin around my eyebrows and nose, the light coating of thrush on my tongue. On my first visit to her she took me by the shoulders and said, "You are not going to die," and that did more for my spirits than the tired wisdom droned at me by all the social workers and therapists and psychiatrists who seemed to spring up around this disease like mushrooms after a heavy rain.

She frightened me as well. "This thing can attack you anywhere, it's like diabetes," she said and suggested that I immediately have my eyes dilated and examined. There was a certain commanding, urgent tone of voice doctors used with me now; my regular doctor spoke like this when he paced in front of me and said, "You *must* take these pills for your mouth," and so did the normally relaxed, courteous Asian ophthalmologist who turned rigid and said, "You have to bathe your eyelids with baby shampoo twice a day." I followed all their directions slavishly, as I had done my whole life with doctors. I had been raised that way.

It was strange to be recognized at the clinic now, on the elevators, in the hallways, in the waiting areas and at the reception desks. I had come the full round, I supposed: I had started out feeling like an exact, highly specified individual in the privacy of my pediatrician's office, then I had slunk unknown and unknowing through huge overburdened clinics, and now here I was, once again an exotic fish, medically speaking, whom everybody knew. I would sit outside the medical building waiting for my ride and wave to all the doctors and staff who were coming and going—the young Turkish ear-man-in-training who had met me in the emergency room one afternoon after a frantic phone call, and who had whisked me through the magic doors into the inner sanctum without making me suffer through the waiting area; the brawny janitor who pushed a sanitation cart up and down the fourth floor hallways; the middle-aged phone clerk who only worked Tuesday and Thursday afternoons.

My presentiment after I had given birth, and the implication I had sensed in the South American pediatrician's words, had turned out to be true: for the rest of my existence, I would be profoundly dependent upon doctors. Anything I chose to do with my life henceforward (provided I was lucky enough to be granted more) would have to be done with my doctors in mind. I would never be able to take a long sea voyage to Antarctica, for example, as I'd once dreamed of doing. I was tethered to the medical community, for better or worse, and my rope could not extend much farther than my physician's reach.

I could not leave doctors, but they could leave me. If I lost a good doctor, I was devastated. It was divorce, utter rejection, even though I knew that most of the time they had perfectly valid reasons for severing the relationship— they had taken a job at another clinic or were going on extended maternity leave or moving out of town. Once I asked a doctor if I could follow her, and I felt exactly like I had when I was fifteen and fell in love with a boy who had made it clear he didn't like me, but in spite of that I still asked if I could be his lab partner in biology. The doctor was mysterious and elliptical, assuring me that she would "be letting her patients know" where she would be; apparently there was some legal reason she couldn't reveal her whereabouts, but I took this to mean that she was avoiding me personally. Somehow she'd found me lacking as a patient, not colorful enough, my symptoms too humdrum

for her taste, my manner too obsequious, my speech too re-
dundant: a terrible bore. I vowed to improve my presentation so that no doctor would ever leave me again.

Painstakingly the groundwork was laid; wearily, we
inched toward mutual understanding. With each doctor I
learned something new about how to be a patient, and
after a few years, I developed a businesslike confidence that
overrode the emotionalism with which I had previously approached medical professionals. I learned to read doctors
the way they learned to read me. I never trusted a doctor
who didn't appeal to me on a certain visceral level, regardless of the credentials behind that doctor's name. If a doctor
yawned in front of me, no matter how innocent the cause, I
lost complete faith and began to search for another. If I
showed up at the walk-in clinic with a cough and the physician on call handed me antibiotics as if they had been jelly-
beans, I avoided that physician in the future, asking to see
someone else if he happened to be on call again. I learned
how to ask for what I wanted, how not to be sidetracked
from my demands, how to make the most efficient use of
the precious thirty minutes allotted to me, how to present
my ailments and complaints clearly and succinctly, without
whining, so that there would be no danger of being mis-
understood. More importantly, I aimed to be respected, and
I came to my appointments armed with research reports
and articles from medical journals and newsletters. I
learned how not to hide things from them: this was just a
waste of time. I learned how not to be timid about expressing even my most trivial complaints, and I learned how to
suppress my natural desire to trivialize my more significant
problems. I learned how to face chronic illness, how to sacrifice the fierce desire to subjugate it for the more rational
and measured wish to co-exist with it. I made doctors my
allies in this crusade for co-existence.

Chapter Four

Penitent, with Roses

The other day, I talked on the telephone to a former lover I had not spoken to for almost twelve years. He was two thousand miles away. After talking to him for a few seconds I realized, with a shock, that he was still alive. He had passed the roughly 4,300 days since we had last seen each other in pursuits much the same as mine—spreading margarine on his toast in the morning, drinking coffee from Styrofoam cups, scanning the newspaper, riding buses and trains, shopping for peanut butter and plastic baggies, watching the t.v. news at night with his feet up on the couch. Every day that I had seen the sun in the sky, he had seen it too. I had quarantined him many years ago, but the relentless fairness of the telephone cable had released him, making a judgment in his favor although I had been speaking of him in the past tense all this time.

I did not have good news. I had telephoned to inform him that I had recently been diagnosed with AIDS. He was not the first man I had called during this post-diagnosis period when, having regained my physical health, I decided to attend to the ethical imperatives that were beginning to press upon me. I wanted to warn these men, not about something that was about to happen, but about something that already belonged to the past; I wanted to let them know the truth I'd stumbled upon while facing backward. The disease highlighted the cyclical nature of life for me and reminded me that there are other cultures that have abandoned the linear approach we take to all things temporal and have devised a more circular view of time itself. We will encounter everything that has happened to us again. I had learned that the glance over the shoulder is a more reliable prediction of the future than the glance into the crystal ball.

It was not so much that I was interested in discovering who had infected me—although of course this might be a by-product of the search—but that I wanted to know who, if anybody, *I* had infected. Although, as a therapist I consulted during this difficult time pointed out to me, even if I were to discover an infected man, there was no way of knowing for sure whether I had infected him. He might have been infected after he knew me, or before. Also, there was no way of telling who had infected whom, although there were acquaintances of mine who at this very moment were wasting precious energy battling over this indissoluble riddle with their partners. The facts were that female-to-male transmission was much more difficult than male-to-female transmission, especially if the female in question was in excellent physical health, which I had been during the period of these love affairs; it was likely that I would get off scot-free, having infected nobody, and having left no trail of bodies behind me. So in one way my telephone calls were gestures only, acts of formal penance.

I decided that I would track down men only as far back as 1985, because that was when I believed I had been infected. Certain symptoms I'd exhibited in the winter of that year—an unusual flu, accompanied by a terrifying full-body rash, were in line with all I had read in medical literature about the symptoms of "primary infection," the body's massively staged immune response to the initial invasion of HIV. I figured that it was unlikely I had contracted the disease any earlier than 1985, both because it was not as prevalent then in the general population, and because if I had been infected that long ago, I would have become sicker much sooner.

So, in the space of a week, I sat down and forced myself to call a list of men with whom I had been intimate in the last decade or so. Some of them were easy to find, requiring only a telephone call to long-distance information, or, in some cases, rummaging through old address books. A few others I found through alumni departments at colleges. One man I could not find at all, despite an Internet search, calls to mutual friends, even appeals to a former landlord. I stopped short of hiring a private detective. I felt a little guilty about this but I knew, for reasons I stated above, that it was unlikely that I had infected him. I let him go, although a bit reluctantly. At this point I had developed a mania for thoroughness which perhaps mercifully masked the emotionalism of my task. I was secretarial, businesslike about this comical and sordid business of reopening old love affairs that had been sealed shut for years.

Speaking to these men was strange, but mostly in a detached, ironic way. Their responses were often funny. Kirk, the self-absorbed older man who practiced transcendental meditation and followed Deepak Chopra, blurted out, after hearing my news, "Thank God I have my support group!" He was somewhat of a hypochondriac and had been tested several times already since he'd known me—I remembered, though, that when I suggested that we use condoms, he had commented that there was no need to fear since only gay men got AIDS. How times have changed, I thought. I did not need to call Ted because he was a friend of Kirk's, and

Kirk, unusually chatty on the phone for a straight man, would dial his number straightaway after hanging up with me. Lee, the gloomy young man with a passion for Dostoevsky, who limped because his right leg was shorter than his left, responded dryly with the automatic sarcasm that was often triggered by nerves, "You don't say." Mark the architect said, "Wow." They all promised to call me back with their test results.

Only one call was truly difficult to make, so difficult that I put it off until the very end, when I could delay it no longer. That call was to Ross, my lover from graduate school twelve years ago. There were various reasons. For one thing, it was during the time I had known him that I had developed the symptoms of primary infection. He had been my only lover in the year we had spent together. I could not imagine that he had HIV—then again, nobody could imagine that I had it either. I was frightened of what I might find out. But, more than that, I had loved him too much; he had wounded me. I did not want to be forced to remember certain things: this seemed unfair to me, not part of the bargain I had struck with my conscience. I would call, relay my news. Surely, after that, my obligations were fulfilled.

Yet, oh hell, it seemed that I was going to be compelled to revisit all my folly, from A to Z.

I found out within a few minutes of speaking with him that he had married a year after our breakup, to the very girl he had left me for. They had two children, older than my little boy. This was hard news for me, a blow to my vanity. Somehow I had wanted to believe that he had left me because of youthful indiscretion or frivolity, not because he had met the woman he had decided to spend the rest of his life with. All these years I had pictured him as a progressively more skillful seducer, someone corrupted by his beauty, incapable of marrying—maybe even mildly debauched—when actually the opposite was true. He was an ordinary husband and father in his mid-thirties.

But I was safe—telephone cable or no telephone cable—because I too spoke to him from within the fortress of marriage and motherhood. I imagined the two of us standing at the outer gateposts of our respective fortresses—pressing our faces up against the chinks in the stone, our view of each other distorted by the necessity of using only one eye at a time—looking out together at the place where we had once been lovers, that shaky, unreliable no-man's land that existed between our two fortresses.

He had been one of the great loves of my life, but I could not remember his voice. "Is this the Ross S—— who went to the University of Michigan?" I asked and he replied it was. I might as well have been speaking to a stranger. When you are madly in love with someone you recognize their voice with your whole body: every cadence, every inflection is instantly registered on each nerve ending. I remembered talking to him on the phone during a week when we were separated and I was not so much listening to his voice as having it dripped into my veins. And now not a single note was recognizable. I found that sad, sadder than the plain fact that he had turned against me and stopped loving me, that he had made a whole life with another woman who was not me, and had children that were not mine. I understood why it had happened, of course—because otherwise I would not have been able to live through all those 4,300 days. Nature itself had protected me by blunting my sensory memory. One can't live at that high, ethereal pitch day in and day out. I could remember that I had loved him and that he had caused me acute pain, but I could no longer feel the love or the pain.

It was tragic. The fact that you could not return, that you had evolved from loving to having loved was devastating.

What then had all that flailing emotion been for? What difference had it made, what use was it? I instantly rejected the platitudinous notion that I had "learned" something from it or that it had prepared me for the more mature relationships I went on to develop in my life. It simply meant that I had at one time felt something very deeply, too deeply, and now I felt it no more. It was a Proustian ache I felt. I had read *Remembrance of Things Past* from beginning to end with passionate attention, and now I identified with poor Swann, who, toward the end of "Swann in Love," laments over his waning love for Odette: "In former times, having often thought with terror that a day must come when he would cease to be in love with Odette, he had determined to keep a sharp look-out, and as soon as he felt that love was beginning to escape him, to cling tightly to it and to hold it back. But now, to the faintness of his love there corresponded a simultaneous faintness in his desire to remain her lover." Later, Swann's love for Odette is referred to as "posthumous."

I could remember the details of our relationship perfectly, although I had no visceral recollection of the man himself. We were both graduate students; I was pursuing a Ph.D. in English literature, and he was working toward his master's in computer science. The first time I saw him was in the community room of the graduate dorm where we both lived. There was some party. He was the most beautiful man I had seen since the man I had noticed on a train in Italy three years before. The man on the train had been a striking American with a head that looked as if it ought to be carved out of bare rock on a mountainside. He was too beautiful to contemplate erotically and he was too beautiful to engage in small talk about the yellow Tuscany hills, and thus I never exchanged two words with him—the most I managed was a bewildered nod of the head. When I got off at my station, leaving the man behind, the pain of having not spoken to him was almost more than I could bear. My failure on this occasion left a kind of psychic scarring: after that, whenever I encountered some desirable person or thing I was always fearful that when the chips were down, I would not really want to act at all, but only to dream. And thus I became even more paralyzed when faced with an object of desire, because I understood my tendency to dream. The man on the train sprang instantly to mind when I met my lover for the first time. The man on the train, I understood now, had been a prefiguration.

And so, not long after I met him at the dorm gathering I pinned a note on his door inviting him to my birthday celebration. It was thrilling to walk away without regretting what I'd done or suffering from a spasm of introspection. To love was to act, to do, not simply to react in turn. I had never before felt so sure of myself. I don't remember if he came to the birthday party, but we soon began to see one another often. One Sunday we went walking in a botanical garden near the university. Leaves were falling on the paths. He picked up one and said to me, "You know, this is the exact color of your hair." I knew then that I existed in his consciousness. It was the first genuine amorous triumph of my life.

He was a few years younger than me, tall, with the grace of certain winged insects in his long legs and arms. Something in him was still unfolding. His well-proportioned limbs were covered with a silky light brown hair; he carried his large hands with a deferential gentleness. He had in fact just gotten used to the span of his body. Every inch had been painfully acquired. He had been on the swimming and rowing teams in high school; he had a robust appetite and piled mountains of rice and noodles on his plate at dorm dinners. "I have to eat a lot or I'll lose weight," he informed me earnestly. He was shyly pleased with the end result of all his growing, in a way that made you indulgent rather than offended.

Often I would arrive a little late at the cafeteria and find him sitting at a table all by himself, except for a girl—usually a freshman—who had tentatively positioned herself a few chairs away, and, nervously flicking at her styled tresses, had dared herself to engage him in conversation. I knew just what she felt like: the exhilaration immediately afterward, and then the long session of rigorous self-analysis in a monastic dorm bed at night: was I interesting? was I pretty enough? what exactly did he mean when he said such and such to me? Waitresses and salesclerks brightened when they saw him. I forgave him because he treated lovely and unlovely girls alike, not seeming to make any distinction between them. His charm was unforced. He even won over my next door neighbor, an angry law student with wild eyes and hair that had been dyed so many times and so many colors that it stood up all around her head hysterically, raw and shellacked. She hated me. "You sure do have a *good-looking* boyfriend," she would hiss at me from the corridors. She liked to knock on my door at eleven o'clock at night while I was typing a paper and insist that I scrub the bathroom that we shared. I usually resisted and a shouting match ensued. But unaccountably he was able to soothe her. Just his presence in a room could make you feel more hopeful about life.

His niceness, in fact, was his second most prominent feature, after his good looks. Twelve years later his essential niceness still shone through the phone cables: the absence of irony, joking, or wordplay, the plainness of his language, made him seem very young. His gentility was natural. Why should he defend himself with wit or humor? He had no need to—everybody loved him.

While I waited for him to visit me in my room, after his session in the computer lab, I would work with uncommon vigor: writing a detailed analysis of the narrative voice in Defoe's *Roxana* or reading a piece of literary criticism on *The Winter's Tale*. Scholarship fueled by erotic energy was a powerful force. In turn, the austerity of my tasks somewhat mitigated the fierce commotion in my breast: on those evenings when I waited for my lover, I achieved a perfect balance, a harmony between heart and mind that I longed to achieve in future love affairs, but never could. After a shy rap on the door, he would enter, his lean, endlessly unfolding body taking up half my room. Nothing we talked about was remarkable. Possibly he told me about his family: his younger sister, whom he adored and worried over (the way Holden Caulfield had adored Phoebe, I was sure), his strange mother who seldom left the house. And other things: an erotic adventure he'd had with a twenty-eight-year-old married woman in an arbor in her garden; his experiences trying out for the Olympic rowing team. His studies, his ambitions (modest, to work for a big company that offered a lifetime of security). Our conversation was anything but fluent. I did not even know how to use a computer, and he had not read the books I loved the most. His benign suburban life was completely foreign to me; my own parents had a more Bohemian take on existence and lived in a house which he innocently described, when he visited, as looking like a "vacation cottage." But my desire for him bridged many gaps. In fact, I did not even notice—until it was over, when I reviewed the whole affair with obsessive hindsight—that we had nothing to talk to each other about.

Talking was hardly what nurtured this friendship, however. We spent many nights on my cramped single bed or his; I never got any sleep, but I had more energy than if I had slept for twelve hours. On Wednesday mornings before the eight-thirty class I taught, I would mount him, both of us breathless, eager, and we would come quickly before I rolled off, threw some clothes on, grabbed my book bag and ran off to the other side of the campus. On those mornings I wouldn't wash, and as I guided my freshman composition students through their paces, I could still feel his presence in my hair, in the secret crevices of my elbows and knees.

Various days and nights stand out in my memory. One morning we made love sitting up in the bed, and did not end our embrace for a long time after we were finished. The campus bells were striking the hour—noon, I think—and the peals were perfectly clear in the cold air. It was one of those brilliant Midwestern winter days. Sun streamed in all around us on the crumpled white sheets. Icicles gleamed on the ledge outside the window. Our legs and arms were entangled. *Remember this moment,* I cautioned myself, and just that second I shifted slightly; there was a cramp in my legs. Perhaps it was the shifting that served to imprint the memory indelibly. In any case I never did forget it. To this day I can hear the bells, and feel the warmth on my lower spine where the sun was hitting.

Foreboding, I discovered, was an inevitable component of a love affair. One day I was watching him as he changed a light bulb in my friend's room—he was so tall, he could accomplish this task by merely standing on his toes and stretching out his hand. He was always helpful like this, with small, practical things that you could not do without. He would come over in a moment if you called him with some little request. I sat staring at his elongated body, the graceful arcs he was creating as he unscrewed the bulb, and suddenly a chill came over me and I thought: *someday there will be an empty space that he used to occupy.* Not

simply nothingness, but one step up from that, absence—
that was the crux of this strange presentiment. Sitting there
cross-legged on my friend's rag rug, I foresaw the future. In
that moment I was bitter—it would have been better for
him never to have occupied that space than to leave such an
abysmal gap. He saw that something was wrong and he got
down on his knees and began to kiss me; in a short while,
the warmth of his mouth called me back to the here and
now, where all was well.

Looking back I believe that he did love me, even if it was
only the temporary and limited love that a young man of
his age and experience could offer. He was always sincere.
One night—he had gone home for the weekend to see his
family—he woke me at three A.M. sounding frightened.
"Are you all right?" he asked. "I had a terrible dream
about you—I dreamed that you were sick or injured or
something." The next morning he cut his visit short and
drove back to me, battling a snowstorm all the way. He
was nearly killed himself when he lost control of his car on
the ice.

He *was* clairvoyant; later on in life I *was* hurt, badly, in a
way that neither of us would have expected. He had
dreamed about my peril a decade too early, that was all.
He was not by nature a fanciful or emotional type, and so
the dream was unusual for him. Perhaps he had gotten
trapped in some kind of psychic interference, had inter-
cepted a message not meant for him at all. Perhaps, also, he
was dreaming of our breakup, which was just around the
corner.

Who knows why some love affairs progress and some
end? I do know that it is often surrender or resignation that
fuels their permanence. Sometimes the urge for one or both
parties to move forward, to move along, is simply too powerful to resist and so they separate. In any case, it is just as

Shakespeare said: men have died and worms have eaten them, but not for love. It is much more likely that you will talk to your lover twelve years later on the phone and not recognize his voice. Is this preferable to dying of love? I don't know.

He returned to school after spring break—which we had not spent together on a trip into the woods of the Upper Peninsula, as I had hoped—distant and distracted. He made excuses not to see me; we were together only two or three nights of the week. Then I confronted him: it turns out he had slept with his old girlfriend over the vacation. Not long ago—a short while before he met me, it turns out—they had been talking about marriage. Did he still love her, I demanded? He didn't know. It was the worst of all possible answers. I was hurt and also confused: this was the first I'd seen of anything flighty or unstable in his nature.

Made uninhibited by grief, I allowed an impulsive friend of mine to intervene for me. She emerged triumphant after an hour or so in his room and informed me that he was distraught and contrite. He had wept. "Do you want to lose her?" my friend had asked and he had sobbed, "No, no." And she had commanded him, "Do the right thing, then!" She was that sort of woman. The next evening there was a knock on my door; I opened it and there he was, penitent, with an armful of red roses.

I felt in that moment that I had conquered him at last: didn't the roses prove it? He looked pale and worn out from his day of repentance; for the first time since I had known him, his looks seemed to be waning. This too seemed to me to be proof of my dominion over him. We discussed everything; he would tell the girl he was through with her, that he was with me now, and that *we* were going to be married. I arranged the roses in the kind of cheap glass vase you always find in dorms and the next morning I walked out of the door an engaged woman. I had never considered marrying him any time soon—I had several years of difficult scholarship left before I would earn my doctorate, and I was shy of matrimony because I did not think I could manage being a wife and a scholar at the same time. But to him it was an all or nothing proposition; he simply assumed that marriage was the natural flowering of romance—that was the way he had been brought up—and I was unwilling to disturb this notion with any more radical suggestions, engendered by reading George Sand and Colette and Simone de Beauvoir and other dangerous female authors. I was terrified that if I did not agree to marry him, he would turn around and marry someone else and I would lose him. It turns out my instincts were quite sound on this issue: he was a young man looking to be anchored, and it was only a question of what harbor he would come to rest in. After our breakup I spent many more years as a single woman, while he got married in a great hurry. But that came later. That night I agreed to become his wife and to all which that implied to a young man of his upbringing—to follow him to his home town, to give up my studies, to have his children. In short, complete surrender. It was a small price to pay, I thought, for absolute possession of another human being.

As for the roses, I pressed the petals between the tissue-thin pages of the first volume of the gargantuan *Norton Anthology of English Literature.* Many years later as I was packing books during a move, I found the petals; they fluttered out, withered but still whole. Immediately, I felt seared again by the humiliations I'd undergone so long ago. I had kept nothing else that had come from my former lover—or so I thought. Just recently, while inspecting my son's toybox, I was surprised to identify a small stuffed bear that he had given to me. It had once been a cherished object—I had loaded it with a symbolism much too weighty for it, just like the roses—but, surprisingly, I felt no desire to get rid of it. I wondered how it had survived the great purging. I felt rather tender toward it. My little boy liked to feed it cornflakes and rock it to sleep: who would ever have suspected that the bear would end up like that? I let it be. Inanimate objects have a whole history of their own that we must respect.

Our reconciliation did not last long. One day about a month later he sat in my little room and told me that he had met somebody else. Not the girlfriend back home—a new girl. He was in love with her. I shouted as if I were warning someone about danger and then I threw a book at him. It missed, clattered to the floor. I began to cry without restraint.

"Why?" I asked, "Why? Why?"

He looked as upset as I was—his large gentle hands clenched and unclenched pointlessly, as if trying to get hold of something. What I wanted to know so desperately was why he loved the other girl better than me, but of course there was no answer to that question. He hardly knew himself. I tried to reason with him—I pointed out that he could not possibly know this woman as well as he knew me, that he was being *disorganized* (I think I actually used this word). And I sobbed and demanded, "Well, what was it about *me* you fell in love with? Think about that!"

He fumbled, young boy that he was, held his hands palm up and replied, "I don't know . . . I mean . . . you have such pretty green eyes . . ."

I sobbed even harder at this answer. It was the worst sort of betrayal—almost as bad as his infidelity. To think of someone describing *me* that way—as just some girl with pretty eyes. To think that he would remember me that way—to think that the whole story began and ended with a pair of green eyes.

(I have since learned that no man would ever be capable of answering the question I put to my lover to my complete satisfaction. I spent years defining love as recognition, the way Rochester and Jane Eyre recognized one another, their essential selves revealed plain as day to the Other who was able, at last, to decipher the cryptic code. But this was not possible outside of literature. I gave up on it. I learned to be satisfied with the beautiful eyes answer.)

I pressed on. "Why?" I kept begging him. "Why her and not me? *Why don't you want to marry me?*" I was not through humiliating myself yet. Sometimes you just have to go the full length. I had been hesitant about marriage, but in my wild state I convinced myself that our marriage had been foreordained, that it was heretical to suggest otherwise.

I pushed him so much he finally found an answer. "Well, you . . . you don't really live in the real world, do you . . . I mean . . . you read books all the time . . . that's all you think about . . . this girl, she—well, she's more . . . well, it's hard to explain."

I wished that I had stopped at the pretty eyes. This was far crueler. He had touched upon my secret fear about myself—the fear that I was not "normal" and did not fit in, that there was some hidden aberration about me, although I strove arduously to conform in all outward appearances. My acquisition of this beautiful and ordinary young man had seemed proof of my success. But he had ferreted out my secret—I "did not live in the real world." Maybe it was as obvious as the nose on my face, and it was all the more mortifying because I had been turning cartwheels trying to disguise it.

I did not live in the real world, so I'd lost him: years later those words still had the power to shame me. Yet I wondered if he would now reconsider his judgment of me. What was AIDS if not the real world? You couldn't get more concrete than that. The virus had carried me farther into reality than I had ever wanted to go, and farther than he would have wanted to go too, I guessed, from his comfortable two-story suburban home, with its remote-control garage doors, central air conditioning, and enclosed patio. I felt a pang of envy for the safe life he had chosen for himself. He had married early and cleaved to a more circumscribed life than I had led; it was entirely possible that I had had more lovers than he. If I'd married him I might have been safe too.

Of course, I realize now that he was right about us. Young and bewildered as he was, he had hit upon the truth. We were not suited for each other in a matrimonial sense. I understood when I'd grown up a little more that what he'd meant was that I did not live in *his* real world. For some reason I had aspired to his real world, but he let me know that it was not appropriate for me. I suppose in some ways he saved me from a lot of unhappiness—he knew, although I didn't, that if I had not been able to live in his real world, then I would have been miserable. Hence, we did not belong together. His arrogance was monumental but innocent.

So the love affair ended, almost as abruptly as it had begun. He tried to be kind, which made the whole thing even worse. After the school year ended and I went home for the summer, he called me once, to see how I was doing, but I said, "I never want to speak to you again," and for roughly 4,300 days after that I kept to my word.

That was when, as I have said, I bludgeoned my way back into his consciousness with the bad news about my health.

What a strange disease this was, I thought: it plucked people out of time and inserted them, all out of context, back into your present life. It scrambled the book of your past. Lives not your own may have been affected by your actions long ago, and yours was affected by theirs. My son did not have AIDS, but his life would be profoundly influenced by a man his mother had sex with many years before he was born. I thought of my lover's children, picturing them long-legged and fair-skinned like himself, wielding Nintendo controls, yelping in one of those plastic kids' pools in the backyard, lazily dumping a clod of fish flakes in a goldfish tank, pouting before a neatly drawn chart on the refrigerator listing their daily chores. Their lives were shadowed by *me*—their father's English major ex-girlfriend. Whom he did not tell tales about, because she was his second-to-last woman, and he remembered her too well. She was not his type, but she'd nicked him. They had never heard of me. And how could they comprehend the idea of a retrovirus which established itself in your most intimate cellular parts, biding its time, quietly reproducing, until one day it stormed the barriers and yanked you backwards out of the present tense? A truly innocent mind could never embrace the concept of AIDS.

A week later my ex-lover called me back; this time my heart really was pounding when I heard his voice. I thought of the mysterious rash that had surfaced one morning when we were in bed together. Was there the slim possibility that my quest, undertaken more to appease my moral self than in any hope of a solution, might produce an answer after all?

"I'm fine," he told me. "I tested negative."

"I'm so glad, so glad to hear that." So my search had led to a dead end, just as I had expected. None of the other men I called bothered to call me back; I took this to mean they were negative, but still, the whole enterprise was clouded by uncertainty. The "primary infection" might not have been so primary after all; perhaps I had been infected years before, and the rash was another sort of manifestation of the disease, or perhaps the rash was entirely unrelated to HIV. The foundation on which I had been building my assumptions had proved to be unsound.

There was an awkward pause in our conversation.

"You're very brave," he said finally.

"Brave?" I wondered whether he meant I was brave to call him. "Oh, you'd be the same way," I demurred. It was the only response I'd found to be truly serviceable when people complimented my courage.

"No, I wouldn't. I'd probably fall apart. Last year my little girl broke her arm and I was a basket case."

"Well, your wife has been brave. I guess this must have been awful for her, I'm sorry."

"Well, well, she had a bad week, but now it's fine. Don't worry about us. I'm sure you have plenty of other things to worry about."

His decency was untarnished by the years. For the first time I strove to imagine what he looked like now, this good human being. My lover in his mid-thirties. Was he still handsome? Still lean, or had he gotten a bit soft? And his beautiful hair? I hoped that time had dealt with him fairly, as fairly as he had always dealt with others.

"What will you do now?" he asked me. "Keep on looking?"

I paused, because I had not even asked myself that question yet. "I don't know. Would you?"

"That depends."

"On what?"

"On how badly I wanted to find out."

"I may have already found it out."

"That's good, then." He sounded happy for me. "What did you find out?"

"That I can't ever find out. That maybe finding out isn't the point."

"What is then?"

"Who knows?"

He laughed. "Okay, if you say so. You're getting way above my head here."

"Anyway, I don't think I'm so interested in finding out anymore."

"Really?"

I wasn't sure if I was sincere.

"You take care of yourself," he said to me gently. "Whatever you do."

I promised I would. We said goodbye to each other without much regret, I think, that we were unlikely ever to talk to each other again. I wondered what I would have lost in my life if, goaded by the memory of the beautiful American man on the Italian train, I had not forced myself to capture my lover's attention, and thus to embark on a love affair. Perhaps it would have been better not to have acted, after all, since what remained was only the empty hull of my love, not the love itself. I felt cheated by the past; it was forever elusive, just as Proust had so eloquently asserted.

That split second in time, would I ever pinpoint its location? No. I decided that I was through dredging up old lovers; there had been a time to do that, and that time was over. It was time, now, to look around me a bit, at the new world I inhabited, and to discover my place in it.

Chapter Five

Who We Are

Of the 33.6 million people worldwide who are living with HIV/AIDS, 14.8 million are women. Six-point-two million women have died since the epidemic began; during 1999 alone, 1.1 million women died all over the world. Women are becoming increasingly afflicted by this disease, not only in developing countries, where 95 percent of the world's population of the HIV infected live, but also in the western industrialized nations of Europe, Canada, and the United States. For the past twenty years of the epidemic the American image of an HIV infected person as white, gay, and male has held strong, but it is gradually being refashioned to reflect the changing face of AIDS in this country. The media and educators are doing their part, but Americans cling fondly to their original beliefs. And from a purely statistical point of view, they are accurate—cumulative AIDS cases in the United States, as reported to the Centers for Disease Control through December, 1999, total 733,374; 609,326, or 82 percent, are men; 124,045, or 18 percent, are women. But when you take into account that the heaviest population of infected women falls between the ages of 25 and 39—prime childbearing years—the statistics begin to look more frightening. The more women who are infected, the more likely they are to pass HIV along to their children, either while in the uterus or through breastfeeding.

Unfortunately, in the United States the disease among females seems to be divided along racial lines. Of the infected women in this country, 71,089 are African American, more than half of the cumulative total for females—a staggering figure, considering that black women account for a much lower fraction of the total population. In African American populations, there are few households that have not been touched by this disease. As for other ethnic groups, white women rank second with 26,960 cases; Hispanic women follow with 24,800 cases. Asian and American Indian women represent a tiny percentage of the total cases.

I am one of these 26,960 white women. I represent a minority, although I occupy a place in the dominant culture, speak the dominant language, and belong to an ethnic group that has traditionally dominated and subjugated other ethnic groups, often whole nations at a time. I am not surprised to find myself an anomaly; it seems to suit my particular psychological make-up. Being a white woman with HIV in the United States, a white Jewish woman at that, puts me in a unique position.

It's a lonely place to be. I discovered after my diagnosis that I had very little community, especially if I wanted to scrape together a community out of women who fit my demographic specifications. I soon abandoned that idea, and began to look for women, any women. At first I had no idea who these women might be or how I would find them. A gay man who lives in the Castro district of San Francisco can literally walk down to the corner drugstore and strike up a conversation with two or three other HIV infected men. In my case, you've got to dig down a few layers to find anybody. The search is even more difficult because so many women—especially white women like myself—are in hiding. They are trying to "pass" as normal, negative folks, the way fifty years ago light-skinned blacks in this country often tried to pass as white.

I am ambivalent about this community too: do I really want to belong to it? I am loath to be counted among the ranks of infected women. I would rather identify myself in any other way—as a writer, a mother, a wife, anything other than an HIV infected woman.

Still, I want to know who else is out there. I begin to long, after a year or two, to relax among other females who know exactly what I'm talking about when I mention "viral load" and PCP. I'm curious as to whether I'm capable of belonging, after a lifetime spent shunning groups. So, with some reluctance, I participate in a retreat offered by an organization called WORLD: Women Organized to Respond to Life Threatening Diseases. Twice yearly, women from all over the United States and occasionally other countries gather in the Bay Area's famous northern wine country.

November, 1998. San Francisco. 9:30 A.M. on the corner of Van Ness and Fell.

The bus is late, of course. A black woman wearing a striped wool cap and smoking a cigarette informs me, "Oh, it was held up in Oakland, it's going to be forty-five minutes, maybe, before it gets here." There is a small group waiting and it swells as the time passes. The sidewalk is littered with our suitcases, portable radios, small ice chests containing medicines that must be refrigerated, packs of cards, oxygen tanks, board games. Three women stand in a group at the curb, smoking, laughing raucously, sharing doughnuts or muffins. "Man, I am *ready* for this," says a pretty woman with a vivid face, high cheekbones, long hair in dreadlocks. "I am going to *party*." Another echoes her,

"Shit yeah, I'm going to have me a good time." Stomping their feet, waving their heads, energy crackling from the palms of their hands.

I am heartened that these women are regarding this trip as an opportunity for revelry. I am always glad to see others in my situation who are enjoying life. I say to myself: See, it's not all that bad. We're just like anybody else, getting excited about a trip.

There is a flurry of excitement as the women run back and forth to the drugstore across the street to buy cigarettes and chewing gum and soda, or to the bakery down the block, or to the bathroom in the building behind us. "Don't you let that bus go without me now!" There is a half-whispered conversation between the smoking women; I pick up a few words. "Nellie . . . didn't you hear?. . . Her boyfriend in jail again . . . and that girl is sick, honey . . . been in the hospital these last two months."

Two women in wheelchairs introduce themselves: Joanne, square, chinless, with tiny eyes and a flat forehead. A thug's face. She has long sparse reddish hair that an attendant, standing behind her, is combing and re-braiding. The other, Martina, is younger, smaller, and softer, with brown moist eyes that seem filmed over. Next to her chair, the paraphernalia of the oxygen-deprived—tank, tubing, carrying case. Both are chain-smokers, dropping their ashes on the sidewalk, directing their unflinching gaze into the middle distance. Joanne converses with me, but Martina is not as accessible. What comments she does venture fade before she reaches the end of a phrase. The two women have an air of not being fooled by the promise that a bus is coming: if one comes, they will board it, if one doesn't, they won't. They've been thrown together by accident but out of this accident they have formed a tough and indomitable partnership. I think of Vladimir and Estragon.

The two women exchange terse comments about the time, the weather. When the attendant finishes braiding Joanne's hair she says, "Thanks, honey. Feels a lot better now." Then she looks at Martina and says, "Did you take your pills yet?" Martina says, "Five more minutes." Joanne says, "You always say that. You better take them." Martina: "I have to take them with food." Joanne: "So get a doughnut." Martina: "I don't like doughnuts, too sweet." She has a small, petulant air. Joanne, soothing, says, "Eat a bagel then."

I strike up a conversation with a garrulous woman named Nikita who says this is her first retreat also. "Oh, girl, I'm so glad, I thought I was the only one." Nikita looks to be about forty; she has long skinny legs and wears pink sweat pants that sag off her boyish hips. Her skull is small and narrow, and her hair, twisted in tiny cornrows, unfortunately accentuates the purplish-black splotches of acne on her skin. There is something so vulnerable, so exposed about her delicate head and bad skin, that I want to throw a scarf around her or adorn her with a fancy hat. But she does not seem to be aware of her exposure; she talks freely, touching me on the arm, illustrating her remarks with robust gestures, her long fingers and blunt nails distracting me with their whirling course through the air. I gather that my nagging sense of impending danger for Nikita, or at the very least my self-consciousness for her sake, is entirely my own problem, and I try to master it and listen to what she is saying.

Nikita got out of jail six months ago—possession, dealing—and now she lives in Phoenix House, a shelter for women struggling to overcome many kinds of addictions.

"It's okay, you know, but I have to share a room with four other women and let me tell you some of them have some *nasty* habits. They dirty, you know? One next to me don't take a shower for three weeks at a time, can't nobody make her, I think the resident counselor called her in ten times about it but shit you can't throw a sister out of that place because she don't shower. Lord, I got a look at her toenails the other night and I thought I was going to lose my supper! 'Cause even in jail I was real fastidious about my personal hygiene, you know? I took a pride in it; braided my hair once a week, wouldn't let it get to look like a rat's nest. So filthiness don't sit well with me. That's something you can do something about. All the rest, maybe you don't have control over, but you can still be clean. I says to my social worker, 'Dolores, I need a break from that Phoenix House or I'm going to go crazy,' and so she told me about this thing and now here I am."

Nikita asks me if I've ever been in jail. "No," I say. I am a little embarrassed by this answer.

She considers this for a moment, and goes on. "Well, you don't want to go there, let me tell you. You stay away from there. They don't even let you take your medications regular. Know what they did? They kept them locked up in this office, like, they call it the pharmacy, but, shit, it ain't no pharmacy, it's just one of the wardens running it and parceling the stuff out after it gets shipped in from the outside. Half the time they don't even know what they givin' you, some of the sisters got the wrong drugs, and I told 'em, I said, 'Honey, you supposed to be taking those pink pills, not those dark blue things.' Wasn't for me some of them be dead or crazy from takin' somebody else's pills. And they don't even let you take the drugs to your cell, every day you got to go out and stand in line, sometimes for an hour or more, just to get your dose. It don't matter what time you're supposed to take them, either, you got to go the times that warden decide to open his pharmacy. So let's say I got to take a pill at three? Well, it's just too bad, 'cause the pharmacy don't open until six. So most of the time I just skipped that three o'clock pill, and *that* ain't good for your health. Doctor I have now though says she's going to get me back on track."

The bus comes. Joanne and Martina wait contemptuously as the driver fusses with lowering the stairs, so they can wheel on. Everybody takes a last puff and smashes their cigarettes on the curb. We all board; some of the women cluster together and begin to laugh and play radios and tape recorders. I find a seat to myself. I am glad: I do not want to talk to anyone else right now. I know I will have to be sociable all weekend, giving of myself in a way that sometimes saps my strength, sometimes gives me an electric jolt of energy—I never know which reaction to expect. For the space of this two-hour drive, I need to gather myself into myself, folding all the layers carefully, like origami.

We arrive at the lodge, a simple but charming wooden structure surrounded by forest and pasture land. There is a courtyard with a fountain near the main entrance, and, alarmingly, a statue of the Virgin Mary on the lawn. Just what we all need, to be confronted by virginity (and hence, purity—spotless blood) at this juncture in our lives. The lodge serves as a religious retreat for groups varying widely in their spiritual practices; there is a whiff of Zen Buddhism in the hallways; the warped wooden floorboards of the lobby are worn by the prayerful feet of Jehovah's Witnesses; and there is a lingering scent, in the closets, in the meeting rooms with their brown folding chairs, of Mindfulness Meditation seminars, Jesuit priests, and Quakers. It's not unpleasant.

I am assigned to a room with three monkish beds covered with rough yellow blankets. None of the doors have locks. As I enter, an anxious-looking Caucasian woman emerges. "Where are the bathrooms? Have you found the bathrooms?" She is thin, pretty, at her nerves' end. Probably in her late thirties or early forties, with big brown eyes. She wears red sneakers. Her name is Mandy. Together we scope out the showers (they look like they're made out of tin) at the end of the hall, and the tiny closeted toilet. Mandy says, "Oh my goodness. Well, I hope my stomach doesn't act up tonight."

We eat lunch in a refectory, buffet style. Excitement ripples through the line; we jostle each other. Food, free food, is cause for celebration. Never mind the nausea and diarrhea and stomach cramps. We are served black-eyed peas, cornbread, meat loaf. Several of the black women whoop with joy.

There is a game—we are all wearing stickers, we have to find the women who are wearing the same sticker and share a table with them. I am a purple butterfly. I sit at a table with Martina and Joanne; they eat solemnly, glancing from side to side, as if they fear someone is going to cheat them of their portion. Eve is another butterfly. I have seen her before at educational seminars and the quarterly meetings of an organization I belong to. She is an activist; she forms women's groups, has started a women's treatment information newsletter, speaks and lobbies on behalf of people who cannot speak for themselves. She is just thirty, a tall girl from Atlanta, wearing glasses and loose clothes. I know her story because she has published it: infected at nineteen, married a few years later to a man she met while working toward policy changes in Washington, D.C., an amicable divorce, the move to San Francisco to help establish advocacy programs. She is here as an educator at the retreat. She is so understated you don't notice her beauty at first glance, but she is the kind of woman you look at twice, then three times, and each time you look, you discover a little more. Hazel eyes and seamless ivory skin. A voice that is always in excellent tune. Hers is an authentic beauty: she draws from the deep well of grace within her. But I notice the shadows in her cheeks, the slight sunkenness. The oversized sweater probably hides the thickened waist. These are the signs by which we know one another.

I tell her I have heard her speak and I ask whether she is still chairing the woman's organization she traveled here to form.

She pauses, considering her answer. "I moved back home. I thought it was time to start giving something to myself for a change. But I'm still active down South. They need me more down there, actually. We take it for granted how many services we have here . . ."

"So you're not really resting that much after all?"

She laughs. A slight southern drawl penetrates the educated patina of her voice. "Way-ell—no, I guess not."

After lunch, our first meeting as a group. We are eighty-five in number. The woman who launched WORLD, the organization that sponsors this retreat, stands up to introduce herself. Her name is Eleanor, and she shares with Eve the modesty, lucidity, and unswerving focus of someone with a calling. Ten years ago, Eleanor started a newsletter from the basement of her sister's house, aiming to disseminate vital treatment information, support, and education to women who were desperately in need of some connection; now the newsletter is internationally renowned, and Eleanor is the executive director of a busy organization that caters to the needs of HIV positive women all over the Bay Area and beyond. Both of these women are natural leaders, although I wonder whether this is a faculty they always exercised or whether it manifested itself after calamity struck. Was Eleanor the president of her high school debate team, did Eve chair the prom committee? No, I cannot see them doing anything of a lesser order than what they are doing now. I decide they have been chosen, as Joan of Arc was. Swiftly, and with perfect aim. Regret stabs me: I am only a writer, and hence a perennial spectator, a little wily, a trifle reserved. I am miserly with my energy and time: they spend it all, go into debt spending more than they have, all for selfish types like me.

Eleanor has straight brown hair parted in the center, a sturdy body, and a pleasant, approachable demeanor. Her face reminds me of seventeenth-century Dutch paintings of women in kitchens doing some humble task—kneading dough, taking buns out of the oven, spinning flax. All she needs is a white pointed cap. I know her story also: positive fourteen years, married for twelve to a negative man, her college boyfriend. Her health has remained excellent; it is possible she is the genuine article—a long-term nonprogressor. We all boast that we are, of course. It's a forgivable vanity: "Oh, I've been positive ten years and I've never been sick for one day, I'm sure I'm a long-term nonprogressor. I'm going to see if they want me for that study they're doing at the NIH." Eleanor herself never boasts; she is half-ashamed of her twelve hundred T-cells. You can't give them away, after all. If she could, she would. Three years ago she and her husband decided to conceive a child and now they have two-year-old twin girls, both healthy.

Eleanor tells us some of the house rules. "Methadone will be kept locked up in my room. Please register with me after this meeting if you are using it. We'll need to see a physician's recommendation and permission also."

She asks us each to state briefly why we came to the retreat. The women start at her left and go around the circle.

"To meet other women."

"To get away from my kids!"

"To find Jesus again, oh yeah, I need to reconnect, baby, it's been too long. I been clean and sober now eighteen months and I need his help to stay that way and I'm hoping I can find him again here!"

(A chorus of approval: "You go girl!" "You'll find him!" "You just hang on!")

"I just need some sleep."

"To meet other women."

"My boyfriend is driving me crazy!"

"To party!"

We rejoin our groups and report what we've learned about each other from a few questions we've been told to ask—who has been diagnosed the longest? who has been most recently diagnosed? who came from the farthest away to be here? who is the oldest? who is the youngest?

Marguerite wins both the youngest and the longest categories. She was infected at birth in 1980; she's eighteen now. She is small—the size of a ten or eleven year old—with shiny black skin, an elongated head, and a fearful manner. The disease has stunted her growth. And orphaned her. So she has been temporarily adopted here by a group of women who cuddle her, feed her sweets, call her "baby" and "darling," and nag her about her medications. She is barely audible, looks down at her shoes as she speaks, and when she's finished ducks back into her group. They close around her like a fortress.

There is a woman from Texas and another woman from Rhode Island.

There is a sixty-five-year-old Asian woman, bundled up to her chin with brightly colored chiffon scarves. Lesions.

An impetuous woman with curly brown hair and bulging

eyes was diagnosed just three months ago, and she's plunging right in, greedy for camaraderie.

Next we have to tell the best joke our group has offered.

A very pretty woman, petite, with slanting aqua eyes, tells a good one:

"You know about the three kinds of sex? Well, there's house sex, room sex, and hall sex. House sex is when you're newly wed and you do it in every room in the house. Room sex is when you've been married a couple of years and you just do it in the bedroom. Hall sex is when you've been married a long time and you pass each other in the hallway and say—'FUCK YOU!'"

Our group contributes one also:

"Okay, so there's this man and this woman going out to dinner, and it's a fancy meal, and the woman says to the man, 'Honey, I hope you know I'm celibate.' And the dude says, 'That's okay, baby, if you sell a bit, I buy a bit!'"

Everybody roars, stamps their feet.

Eleanor stands up on a table to get our attention.

"Sorry to interrupt you . . . has anyone seen Rosita? A little Puerto Rican girl, long curly hair? She's got dementia. I suddenly realized she's not here . . . she could be wandering the grounds somewhere . . ."

Some whispered consultation and then another woman stands up and says, "Rosita's in her room getting an infusion."

Eleanor breathes a sigh of relief. Then she says, "Well, sometimes she gets confused, so if you see her and she looks lost, just take her by the elbow and steer her in the right direction."

Everybody vows to help Rosita, but fear shrouds the room. Of all the demons who stalk us, dementia is the worst. Most other ways of dying we feel we could become

accustomed to, little by little; with morphine and somebody's hand to hold we could get through. It wouldn't be
easy, but we could begin to think of dying as simply a way of
life, our everyday life. Just like other people get up and take
a shower and make some toast, we could be on such habit-
ual terms with our dying. We would prefer to live, of course,
but most of us have reached the point where we understand
that we *are capable of dying* if called upon to do so. But
death from dementia? Never. It's unthinkable. Even the
most callused of us recoil. I pray that the gods are not planning a little poetic justice number—I live by my mind, so I'll
lose it. Like a painter who is blinded by CMV retinitis. Are
the gods this clever, or this literary? Let us hope not.

Resolutely, we get back to our jokes.

Before dinner I venture to participate in a "spirituality"
group held in the chapel adjoining the lodge. My mood
ranges from mild to moderate skepticism. I do not trust the
word "spiritual," it's too slippery, I can't grasp hold of it.
Once upon a time it had a very strict definition—belonging
to the world of the spirits; i.e., ghosts, the undead, et cetera.
But its definition seems to have ballooned to include so
many different kinds of things (like the word "relationship," which I also distrust) that I can really find no meaning in it at all anymore. There is some connection to religious yearnings. Yet it only has a loose connection to
organized religion; in fact, there are many people who
claim to be atheists who also claim to be deeply "spiritual."
I find this puzzling.

However, I do understand that the culture of the HIV infected revolves, almost by necessity, around affirmation, re-
generation, renewal. The body is diseased, so we must look
beyond that, to something that remains inviolate; we must

discover, some of us painfully, our souls. And this is a disease many of us must live with for years, so we absolutely need to develop our higher natures in order to get by. I'm curious and willing to be open-minded. I remind myself that I am new to this culture and that therefore I have no right to judge it until I know more about it. As a newcomer, I still haven't found my place yet. That's why I'm here, to learn and to fit in. Still, I can't help remembering a book in which a famous HIV doctor recommends that positive people write letters to their virus, asking it politely not to replicate, to live in a peaceful state of dormant co-existence with uninfected cells. I pray that our leader tonight will not require this of us.

About ten women are gathered in a semicircle of chairs around a table which is covered with scented candles, incense, small dolls or figurines that look suspiciously, to my Jewish soul, like graven images. Among the women I recognize Mandy and the vivacious one who was diagnosed three months ago. The leader of this group is a plump woman who calls herself Reverend Marcy. She promises that she will conduct an "exercise to increase our spiritual awareness" using the objects on the table. But first she asks us each to talk a little about our "spiritual identity" and how it has made a difference in our lives, especially in the months or years following our diagnosis.

Has my "spiritual identity" made a difference in my life? I don't know. Two years into this game and, if anything, I feel even more connected to my body than before, more absorbed by it: in my effort to hang on to it at all costs, I find every inch of it precious and worthy of the most slavish attentions, and it is only my sense of social propriety that keeps me from talking about my body in relentless detail to all my friends and acquaintances. I have no time for metaphysics or abstractions.

When I was diagnosed my doctor said to me, "You know, there is a spiritual side to healing also." I wanted to slap him. If I'd had a case of the flu, he would have said, "Rest, get plenty of fluids, and take aspirin." No mention of spiritual healing.

Thinking about it later, I decided to give him the benefit of the doubt: perhaps he only meant that the mind could play a role in the body's recovery. That I was willing to grant. I share, with all of the women in this circle, a fervent belief that we can train our minds to eradicate this disease completely. That if only we can focus hard enough, one day we will wake up and it will have disappeared. It is only a matter of learning how.

Perhaps that is what I am seeking from this seminar—a window into what other women know. Tactical advice.

Most of the women interpret Reverend Marcy's question about their spiritual identity as an opportunity for them to testify about how they came to be here and who they are. I am beginning to understand that testimonial is an important part of this gathering, and of any gathering of people threatened by disease.

I do learn a lot, just not what I had expected.

Mandy starts. Her legs are crossed; one red sneaker taps the floor as she speaks. Her tears come easily; her face crumples like a pale linen napkin. She mentions Narcotics Anonymous in reference to the spiritual component of her life. But she does not focus on the twelve-step program. She talks about her husband, who is negative and cannot bear to hear about the disease or to discuss its possible impact on their lives. He refuses to let her tell any of their friends about her condition, claiming that if people knew about her illness, it might damage his career. "He says we should just act as normal as possible. But I feel sick all the time. I had a case of the flu that lasted two months! I'm doing well on the new meds, but it's hard to keep things under wrap all the time. Plus I live so far away . . . I don't know anyone else . . ." She breaks down.

Mandy is just past the first anniversary of her diagnosis. She's past the raw stage, when all you can do is cry and you're afraid to put off seeing a friend until the following week because you think you might be dead by then. Now she is in the stage when you realize that you may not die immediately and this poses fresh problems: how to live with what you know. And what you don't know. How to keep balanced between the two. It reminds me of ballet class many years ago when I was learning how to execute pirouettes without tipping over: always keep your eyes focused on one point on the wall, and return to that point after each spin. That way you'll never get dizzy.

The woman to my immediate left, Frances, does not cry. Sixteen years ago she was given an unlucky blood transfusion after a Caesarean. She is about fifty; short, emaciated, the skin on her face pleated, a bony jaw. Her ankles are so thin a man with medium-sized hands could circle them with his thumb and forefinger. A Roman Catholic. She speaks softly and tells her story with the practiced economy of the long-infected. "I just got over MAC disease, that was rough. And now they tell me I have heart problems! Congestive heart failure. Well, well, you just keep on going, that's all. I've seen some things I didn't expect to see—my daughter just graduated from college, and my oldest son and his wife just had a baby. So there you go." She makes a modest attempt to address the Reverend Marcy's question about spiritual identity. "I'm very close to our parish priest. I can talk to him about anything. At first I know he felt embarrassed, but now he's used to me."

Another woman is also a Roman Catholic. A former nun. She has dark hair shorn close to her head and burning brown eyes that speak of unholy passions, sexual hysteria, or menstrual torture. A tell-tale air of self-flagellation. Shortly after leaving her order, she was raped. "I have renounced God," she says, her voice trembling. Perhaps it is the first time she has said it out loud. "I no longer have any connection to the Church. I find my comfort in the love of other women . . ."

The woman who is three months into her diagnosis cries readily, eyes bubbling. Her name is Barbara. I like the yellow bandanna she has tied around her head to hold back her irrepressible black curls. She is forty-three years old; after having been married for twenty years, she and her husband decided to take a "break" from each other. While on their break, she had an affair with a man in Jamaica, and soon afterward she discovered the unhappy consequences of her fling. Now she and her husband are reconciled. "I believe that God is going to heal me," she says. "I believe He chose me to go through this for reasons of His own but that He's going to stand by me too. I know I have lessons to learn. I don't know what yet, but I know that it will be revealed to me if I only have faith." (A chorus of "amens.") It turns out that her god is a New Age deity. She goes on about crystals, energy flows, chakras, healing herbs, gurus.

When it's my turn to talk, I feel self-conscious and speak stiffly. I tell the women I am Jewish; I describe, without going into too many details, the ritual of Shabbat that I am trying to establish in my household, so that my child will become accustomed to it. I tell them how important it is to me that my child be raised Jewish. The women look respectful but expectant—surely there must be more to tell? I get the feeling I am not participating well. But I'm too much of an introvert for this thing and I begin to wonder what I am doing here. I falter and fade to a halt. Reverend Marcy comes to my aid by telling me that while in divinity school she met many rabbinical students and she feels a great affinity for Jewish philosophy. I nod, embarrassed.

Some of the women speak for so long that we never do proceed to the interesting objects on the table. Reverend Marcy's true function becomes clear to me—she is a shrink. "Spirituality seminar" is a euphemism for "group therapy."

Without skepticism this time, I attend an evening discussion group of women who have children or are considering having children. This is one topic I don't have any trouble grasping or deriving meaning from. The fact of my own little boy's life, his health, his escape from the virus, seems miraculous to me, a sure proof that there is a divine intelligence at work in the universe. Yet I could easily have had an infected child, especially since I breastfed for eleven months. I am curious about women with HIV who want to give birth. The idea troubles me, from a purely ethical point of view, and yet it attracts me too. Not because I want another child—I don't—but because I love the courage embedded in this desire and the exciting implication that we are entitled to our futures. I want to learn more.

Eleanor leads the group. There are several women who are married and want to have children. One is the pretty woman who stood up and told the raunchy joke. Her name is Katrina; she is married to a man who is negative. He is her second husband since her diagnosis; the first man was also negative. The other woman is a sturdy blonde from Texas with straight hair cut in bangs across her forehead. She is married to a positive man. They have kept the fact that they want to have children a secret from their parents, and from almost everybody else they know.

Her name is Helen. She says, "Well, people look at you funny, you know? His parents love me, we get along just fine. They're glad Sam has someone to look after him. But children? I think they'd drop dead of a heart attack. I mean, I don't even imagine such a thought has even crossed their minds—they probably figured we'd put that out of our own minds. When I mention it to doctors, they lecture me about risks. But so many of them, especially in Texas, don't even know the facts. Lots of folks think it's an immoral act, and that's the end of it for them. I'm just like any other woman who wants a child. I'm no different."

Eleanor tells us the facts: if HIV positive mothers are left untreated, twenty-five percent of the babies born to them will be HIV positive themselves. The other seventy-five percent will be fine. And if you treat the mothers during labor with intravenous AZT, arrange for an elective Caesarean and forgo breastfeeding, the risk is reduced even more. At San Francisco General Hospital, which has a famous AIDS research and treatment division, there has not been a positive birth for two years.

Triumphant facts, but I think to myself, there aren't many people who could easily accept an HIV positive woman who knowingly became pregnant. Even the argument that diabetic women can and do have children will not convince them; they will still think of these women as akin to monsters.

"I know a woman who had a kid and died of ovarian cancer two years later," says Eleanor. "There's just no telling."

Katrina tells us about her courtship and marriage.

"When I came to my first retreat eight years ago, I couldn't believe that I'd ever date again, let alone get married. I'd listen to these women and I was like, 'You mean guys actually go out with you?' Since then I've been married and divorced and married again! After my first marriage I realized I didn't have to take the first man who came along. I could be choosy, I could even reject men if they weren't what I was looking for. I always tell the man up front what the score is. So my husband, when I first met him, I wasn't that attracted to him, and I thought, hey, it'll be easy to get rid of him. After all, I have the biggest escape hatch there could be!" She laughs merrily. "So I said to him, 'Listen, I have to tell you something important about myself.' And he listened and he thought about it a minute or two and then he said, 'Yeah? Is that all?'"

She laughs again and we all join her. Katrina has crisp black hair curling around her face, liquid aqua eyes that tilt upward and are framed by thick black lashes. Hearing her boast about her romantic conquests, looking at her pearly nails, her stylish blouse and well-pressed jeans, I feel a rush of pride and confidence. In spite of everything, we still manicure our nails. We apply eyeliner and mascara, we choose our clothes with care! We dare to be beautiful still.

Katrina's husband wants to have a child as much as she does. But her health is not the best at this time. She has "failed" several drug regimens and her viral load is climbing. She is anxious to become pregnant before her health deteriorates further. Several of us express some doubt about her reasoning process. Wouldn't it be better to wait until her body has stabilized somewhat? Pregnancy takes its own toll on the immune system. If her health is bad, how will she care for a helpless infant?

But she brushes aside our doubts. "For me, life is just not worth living if I can't be a mother. Sure, I could take some new drugs, and maybe they'd work, and maybe I'd live forty more years . . . but what am I alive for, if I can't do what I was born to do? If my life has no meaning, who cares how long it is?"

She has touched a nerve; we are silent, pondering her

words. I am reminded of my little boy's favorite Babar book, in which the royal elephant sighs, "Oh, how long we must wait for our heart's desire!" In the early days of this disease, just staying alive was gratification enough. Now we have the luxury of longing again. And longing, for us, is an act of courage. It's what all humans do, and we do it too. Katrina is right: good "counts," or amazing comeback stories not-withstanding, there is much more to life than the sum of our lab reports.

Some of us are curious about how Katrina will manage to conceive a child without infecting her husband along the way. It turns out the effort is fraught with almost surrealis-tically absurd difficulties. Katrina explains, as delicately as she is able, about the turkey baster method. All of us lean forward, listening eagerly. Katrina is obliged to catch her husband's sperm in a cup; then her husband injects it into her. She giggles as she describes how she must keep her hips up in the air for an hour. "There I am, every frigging night, practically standing on my head!"

A few months passed and Katrina still wasn't pregnant. She lowers her voice conspiratorially, looks nervously around, and whispers that they have made a decision to poke a hole in a condom. "Just a *teeny* hole. You know, just enough to let the necessary material pass through."

I feel mildly shocked, although I don't let on. Eleanor jumps in, as if to catch Katrina as she stumbles across a rocky patch. "Bill and I tried all that crap—the turkey baster stuff, the hole in the condom. And none of it worked. So you know what we did? We had sex the old-fashioned way for a couple of months until I got pregnant. But believe me, it was a long time before I could tell his parents or my parents—or anybody, for that matter—how we'd finally managed it."

"Shit, man, our bodies take everything *in*. Their bodies shoot everything *out*," pipes in another woman. We all laugh. We like being a bunch of raucous women together, talking about sex and bodily fluids and men.

Next we come to Lavinia. She is thirty-one years old and has the most beautiful skin I have ever seen: part apricot, part café au lait, it's a heavenly color. Flawlessly smooth, it has a sheen to it, so that even in a darkened room, you could easily pick her out of a crowd.

Lavinia's story is a sad one. Ten years ago she gave birth to a boy and soon afterward discovered that both she and the child were infected. When the boy was two, she married a negative man. They have a happy marriage, although he would like to have a child with her. But she can't bring herself to agree to this.

"The thing is, if I had another child, chances are that child might be negative because of all they know nowadays about how to prevent transmission. And I think I might feel guilty for Vernon's sake. Like he might think, hey, Mom, how come I'm the diseased one and my baby brother is okay? How come *I* have to take pills and he doesn't? I know he wouldn't really think this at all, but it would always be on my mind. Then sometimes I think maybe my husband wants to have another child because he's afraid he's going to lose Vernon—sort of like an insurance policy. And I can't think that way at all. I refuse to conceive another baby just to even out the score, you know? God gave me Vernon just the way he is and I love him that way. I don't think I could ever love another child as much as I love Vernon."

When I return to my room, I find it much improved after a few hours absence—it has become markedly warmer and cozier due to the presence of two animated female bodies and the friendly untidiness of all our belongings strewn everywhere—sweaters, underwear, pill cases and bottles, a teddy bear, books. Mandy is sitting in bed, buffing her fingernails, and she greets me with affection as if we have already known each other many years. She looks much happier than she did in the spirituality seminar; there is no trace of her former melodramatic mood. She introduces me to our other roommate, Beth. I sit down on my bed and we all begin to talk. There is a nice feeling of cold country air pressing against the windows, just enough to make us want to snuggle deeply under our blankets. Trees rustle outside and a cat purrs on the fire escape. In the room we understand that we are quite safe—not only from the elements, but from viruses and other horrors. At least for these few nights, anyhow.

We swap stories. Mandy goes first.

"My brother's got it too—sixteen years. So when I found out, it wasn't that much of a shock to me. It was almost like I *expected* to get it. Nothing new. We've always been close, even though our lives have gone such separate ways—he's gay, he's wrapped up in that world." She smiles. "So now we call each other up, compare counts, talk about the meds. Our parents, though—*man*—only two kids, both infected. Of course they always thought we were pretty worthless anyhow."

Mandy and her brother ran away from home together when he was sixteen and Mandy was fourteen. Their parents were deaf; their first language was sign language. "They were really mean to us—used to beat us with broomsticks, rolling pins, whatever they had at hand. I don't know why they hated us so much." She shrugs. "Maybe because we could hear and they couldn't? Maybe because they were afraid of what we were hearing?"

When she was sixteen Mandy met her boyfriend and at seventeen she had a stillborn baby. A year later she had her daughter, who is now twenty-five and has a five-year-old son of her own. Mandy is the youngest and most stylish grandmother I have ever known. You cannot read her rough beginnings in any aspect of her appearance or speech—not in her porcelain skin, her expensively cut hair, her long neck or her hand-knit Icelandic sweaters. You would never imagine in your wildest dreams that Mandy and her brother had once lived on the streets, popping acid in Haight Ashbury and sleeping in doorways.

I have a special fascination for people who have remade themselves from scratch. Their lives are so much like fiction, my enduring passion. The difference between what I do and what they have done to themselves is simply a matter of medium.

When I comment upon Mandy's tumultuous youth, she smiles and says, "Oh, I've lived a life." Even the modesty of her response reminds me of certain writers who, when praised for their work during the question and answer period of a reading or lecture, reply, "Well, it practically wrote itself."

I tell my story too. They are sympathetic and ask all the right questions, but they are not too surprised. Here, in this arena, my story is commonplace. I'm comforted by this fact. I am tired of people regarding me as the subject of a tragedy, of the pitying nods and the ineffectual and sometimes insincere offers of assistance. "Your life must be a nightmare," a negative friend once remarked and I resented it, took offense, although he meant only to express sympathy. Only other positive people could understand how you take HIV and weave it into the fabric of your life, creating new patterns as you go along. Women, who have to take care of children and husbands and pets and get dinner on the table and do the laundry, are especially good at putting HIV in its place. We're too busy for nightmares and Greek tragedies.

Now it's Beth's turn. She is a young girl, not more than

twenty-five or so, with a rather spoiled, puffy face and small nervous hands that clutch at her bedcovers as she talks. She hails from Beverly Hills: she dresses simply, in baggy pants and shapeless T-shirts, probably to disguise her background, but nobody is fooled. Her luggage is Gucci. She's the kind of girl who was always protected and taken care of, like me. She still can't accept the fact that something bad has happened to her. I feel sorry for her; I know if she were my age, it would be easier for her, but this is her *youth,* for God's sake. She's about the same age I was when I was infected but, either mercifully or regrettably, whichever way you look at it, I remained ignorant until many years later. Now she's been cheated out of her twenties, those arrogant, delightful years in a woman's life.

She knows who infected her, but he won't admit it. This is driving her crazy. She sniffles. "He was just one of these guys—the type who just sweeps you away. You know, fancy dinners, weekend trips, gifts. I was blown away by him, I thought we'd get married. I didn't know very much about him, I have to admit. I met him at a party on a yacht. This friend of mine, she was engaged to this guy who is friends with the guy who owns the boat, so she got me on. I was all, like, hey, I'm going to meet rich guys, this will be cool. And guess what? I did meet a rich guy! Yeah, lucky me!" Suddenly she pounds her fists into the mattress. Her neck and face are inflamed. "I was so *fucking naive.*"

We murmur comforting words about her youth, her lack of experience.

"Yeah, it was a real brain-fuck . . . He claims *I* gave it to *him.* That slays me. I said that wasn't possible, that six months before I met him I'd gotten a negative test and there hadn't been any men between that time and him. And I tested positive a few months after we broke up. So go put two and two together, okay, asshole?"

He won't talk to her anymore, and she can't get him to admit that he may have had it for years already and not known. She had a tough time even convincing him to get tested. "I tell him, 'Hey, I'm not accusing you of deceiving me. I know you didn't know. All I want is for you to stop putting *me* down, stop making it look like it's my fault. We're in the same boat here. All I want from you is to acknowledge that, okay?' But he won't do it."

She drives her fists into the mattress, then starts pulling at both sides of her hair.

"He's still fucking with my head! After all this time!"

Mandy moves over to Beth's bed, puts her arm around her shoulders, makes shushing sounds, until gradually Beth calms down. Beth is probably about Mandy's daughter's age. We offer all the conventional wisdom at hand: what's done is done. The past cannot be corrected or amended. The man's self-deception is punishment enough in itself. It would be far more productive for Beth to concentrate on her future, and to avoid the mistake of letting herself be judged by someone who is such an unworthy human being.

But although I believe these are the right things to say in the circumstances, I'm not sure if I believe them, not with any deep conviction, anyhow. None of us is ever done with the past. Sometimes we pretend we are. Yet the past is what marked us, and it has the power to madden us too, if we let it, like it has maddened Beth. We all say to ourselves, "If only, on that night, I hadn't . . ." or "If only, instead of this . . . I had done that . . ." We think endlessly about those few seconds in time, out of all the seconds of our lives, which changed us forever. Those few seconds would always be part of the present for us. I think of my fruitless search, the ex-lovers I called, and I am envious, because at least Beth knows when that moment was.

If the man apologized to Beth, the internal dialogue might not stop, but it might be quieted, like turning down a radio to a low volume. We've all discovered our own ways of minimizing that dialogue so we can hear other voices too. But we're deluding ourselves if we think that we can turn our backs on it altogether.

Soon we are all tired and undress for bed. After our confidences, we don't hesitate to disrobe in front of one another. Since I so rarely see any breasts except for my own, I find myself quite curious about my roommates' breasts. I consider the fact that I have probably seen more penises in my life than breasts, and this is somehow funny. I sneak glances at Beth and Mandy.

Beth's breasts are heavy and tubular, with thick brownish nipples. I'm reminded unpleasantly of a cow's udders. My breasts are small and droopy from nursing, no better. But Mandy has great breasts. She is slow to reveal them. While Beth and I simply remove shirt and bra all at once, she makes a small ceremony of it. She lingers awhile in her bra, a dove-gray silk number that lifts her breasts gently higher and shows off the whiteness of her skin. There's a small brown mole on her left breast, near the nipple. The two globes are full yet delicately molded, large yet airy, like some spun-sugar confection. The pink nipples tip upward. She remains naked a few more moments than she needs to be, examining her fingernails, and then she slips a nightgown over her head.

We all sleep very well that night and wake up completely refreshed.

The next morning I attend a seminar about new treatment options led by Eve. A stocky woman with big red glasses and white and black spiked hair takes the empty seat to my left. On my right is a young woman with a full figure. She could be a *Playboy* model. Whenever I shift slightly in her direction, I catch her staring at me; then she lowers her eyes and blushes. The woman with the red glasses stares at me also and says, in a loud whisper, "Can you see? Am I in your way?" I stare straight ahead and reply that I am fine.

I experience the glances they send my way as a slight tingling on my earlobes. I feel quite the femme fatale, surrounded by admirers. I listen to Eve. The woman with the red eyeglasses slips her hand on my thigh. She keeps it there a few moments, her fingers moving in tiny circles; with each circle, she presses more insistently at my flesh. I behave the same way I do when a man makes an unwanted pass at me: secretly I enjoy the compliment but outwardly I act haughty. After awhile the woman removes her hand and the tingling in my earlobes subsides.

Although I'm not a lesbian, the idea of anyone expressing an interest in me sexually is gratifying. Thanks to that woman's hand on my thigh, I feel somehow reconnected to a part of my life I assumed had been severed from me. I feel like a lovely person again.

After lunch, the sun is shining and the air is balmy, so I decide to skip a few seminars and go for a walk through the woods to find the treehouse that has been billed as one of the lodge's attractions. I am the only woman on the trail; a quarter-mile jaunt uphill brings me to a clearing in the woods where a huge oak tree stands, upon which the treehouse has been built. It is an elaborate, beautifully constructed edifice: three tiers, with a wooden staircase winding up through the branches of the tree. A brass railing spirals alongside the stairs. I pause before mounting the steps, enchanted with this spot. The air is still and pellucid: from far away I hear a cowbell tinkling, and in the dry underbrush a small animal rustles. I sniff the pervasive, spicy, evocative scent of eucalyptus, and I crunch some of the nuts under my shoes. I have the wonderful illusion, not hard for me to discover whenever I am in nature, that I have become a clarified version of myself, with my character distilled to its finest points, and the clutter of personality swept away. I simply float above all the usual junk I have to wade through to get to who I am.

So I'm buoyant when I climb. Then I notice that the brass railing is etched with the names and dates of birth and death of many people. The names snake all the way up to the top and I realize, the higher I reach, that they are all men, and that they have all died young. Strange, since this is a women's retreat, that there are no women's names on it. But the treehouse was probably erected long before women began using this ranch for the same purpose many men did before us. I check the dates again—yes, all these men passed away eight or nine years ago. And there's no room left on the railing for more. Now I feel deflated—and betrayed. Nobody warned me that this was a *memorial* treehouse. We can't let our guard down, even for a moment. The sensation of transcendence I have been experiencing in the clearing could be a hint of the transportation effected by death: once you were over there, in a body, but now you are here—a name, a date, an essence, a memory, and an elemental part of the earth.

Only I don't want to be *that* distilled, thank you. I am fond enough of my own jumbly identity not to want to lose it so easily in the anonymity of chemical elements. No matter how much I love nature, I don't want to replenish it with my own body, not just yet, anyhow.

* * *

I think of the first woman I ever knew who died from AIDS, somebody from graduate school. But, of course, this was 1985 and nobody knew what she died from, let alone me.

You would have thought you were looking at a famine victim. You could see the outline of her ribs through her shirts, and even when she wore a wool coat, her elbows seemed to poke through the fabric. Her lusterless hair hung in two limp ropes on either side of her face. She would buttonhole you if you ran into her on campus and catalogue her woes—fevers, fatigue, a general feeling of overwhelming malaise. "Student Health says it's mono, there's nothing they can give me for it. Just rest. But how can I rest? I've got to teach my classes, grade papers. I've got to get at least the first draft of my master's thesis to my advisor by March 1. And meanwhile I can barely drag myself out of bed in the morning, it takes me forty-five minutes to get dressed . . ."

This went on for months. We grew frightened of her, she seemed to bode evil, and we avoided her wraithlike form when we spotted her on the quads, shivering, a black wool cap jammed over her forehead, her gait unsteady, her knees buckling under the load of books she carried in her arms.

Then, one day, we learned from her roommate that she had died. The roommate had found her in the middle of the night on the bathroom floor, gasping for breath, her body burning to the touch. By morning, she was gone—the hospital listed the cause of death as pneumonia. But no twenty-five-year-old woman, without a previous history of respiratory illness, dies of ordinary pneumonia. She died of PCP, the fatal pneumonia brought on by AIDS: I'm sure of that now, although nobody suspected it then. We wrote off her unusual death to the inadequacies of Student Health, and to the eccentricities of the girl herself, who was notorious

for eating only jelly donuts for days at a time, and forget-
ting to wear jackets when the weather got chilly. Anyone
who took such bad care of themselves was bound to come
to a bad end.

And in 1985 I had recently been infected myself. I did
not realize, I had no way of knowing, as I stood nervously
looking over her shoulder for a means of escape while she
recited the ceaseless litany of her aches and pains, that she
was describing the symptomatic stage of the very disease I
was then carrying within my own bloodstream. She was my
future—eleven years later, I would look just like her, my
hair falling out, my skeleton beginning to assert itself, to
mock the precipitous decline of muscle and flesh. "Don't be
fooled," her body seemed to warn you, "Bone is the su-
preme master. It's at the end of everything. Bone is all there
is." For a brief moment, time had been compressed, like a
coil of rope with the two ends touching.

In those days there was no one to identify her illness for
her. There were no women's groups, no women's clinics, no
Eleanors and Eves to mobilize us, to infuse us with courage,
to remind us that we were not alone. There were no *women*
as far as anyone knew. But of course, we were there right
from the beginning. We were just well-hidden. When we
died, we died like my fellow student: in utter isolation, ignorance, and unfathomable fear.

The second night there is a talent show in the large meeting
room where we all congregated the first day. Although all
of us have been invited to perform, there are only a few
white women who choose to take the stage; the majority of
the performers are black. But we all attend the performance, huddling near the stone fireplace, bundling our
chilly skins in extra sweaters, even mittens. I feel small,

insipid, ridiculously intellectual watching these women blaze and stomp across the front of the room.

They don't care about us; they're performing for each other, and for themselves. I think: *if only I could step out of my body, I'm so weary of being myself, dear God.* A lot of what they do is sheer silliness, meant to blow off steam. But some of it is inspired comedy, and some of it is eloquent. I wonder, how do a bunch of sick women find the energy to put on a show? I've heard all of them complaining about sore muscles, bad stomachs, shortness of breath, at least five of them use a cane, one I've seen occasionally in a wheelchair—yet here they all are, vying for stage time.

Tiny Marguerite overcomes her shyness and sings a pop song by a black female singer. It turns out she has a lovely wavering soprano voice and the applause is enthusiastic. She breaks only at the end, giggling and diving back into the arms of all her surrogate mothers. Four women get up to perform a rap song they've written themselves: "Now back off, virus, 'cause you got to fight us, and we ain't givin' an inch/oh no/it's a cinch/we bitches and witches and you best watch out/or we'll give you some stitches." (One of the women is Barbara, who was diagnosed three months ago and who wept so copiously during the spirituality seminar. She's put a baseball cap backwards on her head and in spite of her white skin manages to affect a plausible African American manner. Nobody seems offended by her. She hangs out with the black women during the seminar, feeds on their exuberance, and they tolerate her. I think, like me, she longs to be anyone else but herself right now. Three months out is hard and you do what you have to do to get through. If she needs to be black, so be it.)

A gorgeous statuesque girl reads a poem by Maya Angelou. I've never seen a face built on such a scale as that—the round high cheekbones, the slanting eyes that seem to stretch from her temples all the way to her nose. Sturdy legs that could keep the Parthenon standing for a thousand more years. The poem is about being a woman and in her hands it transcends the somewhat politicized subject matter that grates on paper. I am reminded that poetry was originally sung to enthusiastic audiences. The girl's recitation is great theater—perfect cadences and timing. The audience howls its approval. She's one with the poem and I'm sure Maya Angelou would agree.

The climax of the evening is a parody of a television talk show which is itself a parody of television talk shows—a popular program that people watch in spite of themselves, in order to witness the vulgar spectacle of human beings fighting, scratching, and biting each other on stage. The lesbian with the full figure who sat to my right during Eve's seminar plays the girlfriend who discovers that her boyfriend is cheating on her; she wears a tight white T-shirt, pouts, and thrusts her chest toward the audience. A black woman with a formidable hairdo of spirals and corkscrews plays the boyfriend, managing to look masculine by squaring her shoulders and placing her hands flat on her knees. The Maya Angelou interpreter is the "other woman." The talk show host is played by a woman with a shaved head and a snake tattooed on her arm; she uses an enormous plastic-cast penis as a microphone, which in itself causes wave after wave of hysterics in the audience, especially when she grasps it by the balls and twirls it. "Hey, what are you laughing at?" she cries, pointing the penis at somebody in the audience, and we all laugh even harder.

The players have a dialogue to follow but they soon abandon it for the sheer euphoria of ad-libbing. The talk show host attempts to interview the women but is physically attacked by the "man." The women strut their stuff, entreat the audience to take their side, and end up grabbing each other's hair. The host intervenes, bonking them both over the head with the penis. "If you don't shut up, I'm going to stop up your mouth with this thing!" she threatens.

"Oh, I'm going to pee my pants!" cries an audience member, doubled over with laughter.

It's impossible to hear what anybody on stage is saying anymore. Pandemonium ensues. The actors run into the audience waving their arms and the audience mixes with them, you can't tell who's who, it's like a wild dance, and suddenly the show is over and everybody is bowing, the actors glistening, grinning, and panting.

That night in our room, Mandy tells us the story of her marriage. Three months before her wedding, she was diagnosed. The wedding proceeded exactly as planned—her husband remained imperturbable—and she proudly shows us a picture of herself looking flower-like in a light blue, low-cut dress, a blue ribbon in her hair. She is leaning on the shoulder of a robust, broad-chested man with bushy white hair and a firm chin. He meets the camera head-on, with a challenging frown.

Mandy's face turns melancholy, in spite of the joyful nature of these photographs. "You know, my husband is a good-looking man, he's attractive to other women. Sometimes, when I'm feeling down, I say to him, 'Why'd you marry me, this diseased person, when you could have had any woman? Wouldn't you rather have a normal woman?' And he just gives me this look like I'm crazy. Like if I don't know why he loves me, then he won't anymore. I get afraid. I don't know what I'd do without him. I can't start all over again—I've done that too many times in my life."

We know all too well what she means. We've all started over at least one too many times—the most recent being when we were diagnosed, when we had to start reforging our identities from scratch, realigning our past with our present, and learning to sacrifice the long view. Could we go through that again, would we have the stamina, the psychic energy required to begin yet again? Mandy looks to us for reassurance, but we really have nothing to offer her. What guarantee is there that her husband won't leave her? None. The scaffolding we have all erected for ourselves is heartbreakingly fragile.

It is our last day at the retreat, our last breakfast, and something unsettling happens. We are digging into our meal of pancakes, bacon, eggs, and granola, when Frances, the thin woman with congestive heart failure, suddenly rises from the table, her hand clapped over her mouth. A woman sitting next to her helps her out of the room and into the little alleyway outside. Soon Frances returns to the table, a bit pale and shaken, but still determined to finish her breakfast. She insists that she is not ill.

"Oh, sometimes I just throw up," she says, shrugging her shoulders. "I wasn't feeling sick or anything. It just happens—like a reflex—or sometimes when I cough too hard. Two or three times a week I'll throw up, maybe more."

All of us have put down our forks, but she resolutely spears a sliver of bacon, stares at it hard, then shakes her head and puts it back on her plate.

"Better wait awhile," she sighs. "The worst is, now I have to take the pills all over again. All five of them! Not one of those little suckers got digested. If only I could wait to be sick until after they've gotten into my bloodstream, but I can't time it . . ." She laughs weakly.

None of us dare to ask the nauseating question that occurs to us.

As if she can read our minds, she replies, "Oh, I count them. I know it sounds gross, but I have to. I get a stick or something . . . swirl around . . . it helps that they're bright blue."

She digs in a large handbag under her chair, brings out an enormous white plastic bottle, shakes it, sticks out her tongue at it, shakes it harder, and slams it on the table. "Jesus, I can't even stand the way these things smell. That *medicine* smell, you know what I mean? I can't ever get rid of it, sometimes I think I smell it everywhere."

We all know what she is talking about.

Frances continues, "Well, I've just got to get some breakfast down me. I'm not leaving this table until I've had at least two pieces of toast with lots of butter and five pieces of bacon."

We bring her fresh, hot food, a cup of strong coffee, a tall glass of juice, encourage her and cheer her on. But she can't. Sadly she says, "I'll try again at lunch . . . but I've just got to gain weight, I just have to. I've been through two different steroids and an appetite stimulant and nothing has worked. My doctor says he's going to hospitalize me if I don't put on five pounds by next month . . ."

My own appetite is gone too. I feel as if I will never be able to eat again for the rest of my life. I can predict what will happen. Frances will fail to gain five pounds and she will indeed be hospitalized, and will spend many months hooked up to IVs, subjected to tube feedings, to invasive examinations of her colon and esophagus. She will be violated in hundreds of ways before she is finally allowed to slip away, tubeless.

I walk away from breakfast shaky in the knees. Flesh is all I can think of—how much I crave it. Forget about the soul. That can take care of itself. Flesh is what you want—thighs, buttocks, bellies, breasts—great Rubenesque rolls of it, layer upon layer, each more fatty than the next. That's the only security there is.

It's time to go. The bus is waiting for us, and Eleanor has summoned us once more as a group into the large meeting room. She has asked us all to bring a leaf; she passes around two large ceramic bowls, one empty, one full of colored glass beads. "Drop the leaf in the empty bowl and tell us what you are leaving behind," she instructs us. "Then pick out a bead and tell us what you are taking with you."

She begins for us: "I am leaving behind fear and taking home courage."

We all join in:

"I am leaving behind ignorance and taking home knowledge."

"I am leaving behind isolation and taking home friendship."

"I am leaving the devil behind and taking Jesus with me."

"I am leaving behind suspicion and taking home trust."

"I am leaving behind addiction and taking home strength."

"I am leaving behind bad thoughts and taking home my heart."

When it's my turn, I say, "I'm leaving behind myself and taking all eighty-five of you home with me instead." Everybody laughs and somebody jokes that I'd better have a big apartment. I feel suddenly shy when I see them all beaming at me. I mean what I've said on several levels. As a writer everybody I meet always comes with me—nobody is ever left behind. But I mean it on a literal level as well. I want each one of them—their words, skin, hair, laughter, silliness, and wisdom. I want to be crowded and jostled; I want it noisy; I want to be *attached*.

Chapter Six

Working on the Line

My first call of the morning, after I have settled myself into my booth with a cup of coffee, schmoozed with my neighbor and logged in on the phone line, goes something like this: "I got this roommate. He's drivin' me crazy. I know he's gay. I know he got that thing, that disease. All of them do. Well, we share the same *sugar bowl* in the morning. I eat my breakfast second, after he gets up, and I know he's been putting his spoon in there because he puts sugar in his tea. Seen him drink it that way. Me, I put sugar on my Cheerios. Still, it's the same sugar bowl, ain't it? I ask him, did you ever go get yourself tested? He says no and he doesn't aim to either. I tell him he better get tested, I'm going to kick him out. It was my apartment first. He just laughs at me. Aren't there some laws about that? That he got to get tested?"

It occurs to me, not for the first time during my year of working on the San Francisco AIDS Foundation's HIV/AIDS hotline, how much we rely on subtext to guide us through the maze of human relations. And on this job, our reliance on subtext is even more pronounced. Our ears are pricked for signals: even the most literal among us know how, on some level, to hear beyond what we hear, to sort

meaning from intention, to distill the essence of somebody's humanity. Voice reveals all: social class, education,
sexual orientation, ethnicity, age, emotional and geographi-
cal compass points, assorted prejudices. I find myself cub-
byholing people and not feeling any pangs of conscience
about this, although in "real" life I'd censure myself severely if I noticed myself exhibiting those kinds of biases.
Nevertheless, I'm a good counselor: I'm sympathetic and
patient and I try to accept different points of view without
imposing my own on the conversation.

I guess that this caller is an elderly man who probably
hails from some rural community in Southern California,
or possibly the Central Valley. (The hotline covers all of
California. We get relatively few calls from San Francisco,
although we're based here: I wonder if that's because people in this city are better-educated about the disease, or if it
has simply become such a part of the fabric of their lives
that they seldom think twice about it.) He barely graduated
high school and he worked for most of his life as a me-
chanic or a welder. Something, I'm sure, with metal—
there's a scratchy tone to his voice that I associate with
wrenches and axle grease.

I point out, gently, that not all homosexual men have
HIV. If his roommate is even homosexual, which he admits
he is not sure about. I explain that the virus cannot be
transmitted by casual contact. Before I launch into my
usual spiel about transmission—the three most dangerous
bodily fluids, the three most risky sexual practices, in order
of descending risk—I ask him if he understands how the
virus is passed from one human to another. Mercifully, he
does. Even senior citizens nowadays are spouting that ex-
quisite oxymoron, "safe sex." I describe the delicacy of the
virus, how it cannot survive for long outside the body and
certainly not in a sugar bowl. Then I clinch the argument:

"If it were that easy to transmit HIV, many more people would be sick." He appreciates this logic, but he can't quite let go of that sugar bowl. He asks if there is any way to force his roommate to get tested. I tell him this is illegal. Still, he's not satisfied. "Don't you think *I* should be tested?" he whines. I ask him if he has engaged in any "risky behaviors" lately. "Sweetheart, not since before you were born!" he crows.

Having said all I can say, I wriggle my way out of the conversation. He says goodbye reluctantly, wanting to talk more about sugar bowls and Cheerios and suspicious roommates. I wonder if he feels any better: maybe by a hair's breadth. We are required to ask a few demographic questions before hanging up. He lives in Fresno, he's white, he's seventy-seven years old. His roommate is eighty-two.

Fear is the dominant chord on this hotline. We have labeled people like this man the "worried well," and there are plenty of them out there. I am always amazed at how many people are frightened of acquiring HIV. Ironically, I never was myself, and here I am. Between calls I wonder idly if the whole course of my life would have been changed if I had just learned to be a frightened person. Once we hang up, we often ridicule the "worried well" to our fellow volunteers, as a way of blowing off steam, but sometimes I think they're onto something. The world is a damned scary place.

The under-educated do not have a monopoly on fear. The well-educated "worried well" abound and they are often much trickier to deal with. They analyze, argue, interrogate—they are capable of sustaining lengthy metaphysical discourses about the disease. A woman calls: her voice is crisp, cultured. I guess she is in her mid-forties. Lives in Santa Barbara. Has an M.A. in art history. Gets a weekly facial. She explains she is a bookbinder and that she recently shared studio space with a colleague who is now deceased.

She only recently discovered the cause of his death; apparently the poor man never "disclosed." She is fretting about an Exacto knife they often passed to each other. Could his blood have been on it? Could the virus have passed from the knife into her own bloodstream? Indignantly, she states: "I think he should have told me he had AIDS, don't you? I mean, don't you think I had a right to know?"

I ask her if she ever saw him cut his finger with the Exacto knife.

"No, but . . . well, he could have and I just didn't notice."

"Doesn't an Exacto knife have a very sharp blade?"

"Oh yes, very."

"So if you cut yourself with it, you're really going to bleed, right? I mean, you're probably going to shout. There's no way you wouldn't notice if someone cut themselves with that."

Offended silence on the other line.

I pursue my line of reasoning. "Did *you* ever cut yourself with that knife?"

"Well, no . . . but I may have had a hangnail . . . or a papercut . . . that would provide an opening into the bloodstream, wouldn't it?"

"It's not very probable."

"Yet *possible,* right? Theoretically, if there was some of his blood on the knife, and he passed it to me and I brushed my cut up against it, I could contract the virus, right?"

"Technically, but . . ."

Now she has the upper hand.

"So you're saying it could happen."

"But the virus can't live outside of the body for any significant amount of time. Except inside of a needle. And that's not the situation you're describing."

"If it's in *blood* it can survive, though, right?"

"A little longer, maybe . . ."

"How long?"

"Nobody knows exactly . . . depends on the amount of blood . . . There would have to be a lot . . . Listen, the situation you're describing is extremely rare . . ."

"Well, the world is full of rarities, my dear."

"You could be hit by a bus when you cross the street also."

She's not buying this. "Do you have any *exact* statistics about the possibilities of transmission by this route?"

Invariably, the educated ones all ask for statistics.

Finally, I advise her to get tested if she is really worried. It turns out she was tested, twice, in the last three months. The results were negative.

"But you just never know, do you. I read that the rate of false negatives for the test is very high . . ."

Then there is the woman who has not had sex in eight years. Last Friday night she had a date with a man she didn't know very well, someone she was fixed up with. As they parted at her door, he kissed her. "I don't know what to do," she pleads. "Should I get tested? Is it too soon? I know there's some kind of window period . . ." The urgency and terror in her voice frighten me in spite of myself. I think of all the men I kissed when I was single: who could even begin to count? And if I could turn back time, unkiss them, would I do it? Yes, yes! I think of Romeo: "My lips, two blushing pilgrims . . ." And all the pretty flirtation that follows. What a dangerous subversive that Shakespeare was! How could I ever have allowed myself to be seduced by that poetry—to be seduced into taking up kissing myself!

Struggling to subdue my own panic, I ask the woman if she and her date were engaging in any deep, French kissing.

"Oh no," she says. "I'd never allow anybody to do that. He kissed me on the cheek. But it was right at the *corner* of my mouth, see. I mean some of his saliva could have . . ."

Nowadays, sex and the fear of death go hand in hand. The Marquis de Sade would have had a field day. I despair for the world's dwindling supply of healthy eroticism. If you work on the hotline too long, you secretly want to cheer anybody who tells you they had great sex the night before, no matter how "unsafe" it may have been.

And, as it turns out, I do hear plenty of these stories. At the opposite end of the spectrum from the "worried well" are the callers who are indeed still having sex, abundantly. I get many calls from young gay men who were just children during the darkest era of the plague and have never seen the purple blotches of Kaposi's sarcoma. They go to dance clubs and take a drug called crystal meth which enables them to have sex all night long, usually with several different partners. These men are talking about unprotected anal sex, the most dangerous behavior there is, with the exception of injecting drugs from a used needle. They apologize to me (I must sound maternal to them) but explain that they were so "wasted" they forgot about condoms. Do I think they put themselves at risk? Yes, I say, they did.

"Really? But the guy told me he'd tested negative."

I explain about the unreliability of using the HIV antibody test as a way of determining whether someone is a "safe" sexual partner. Most people don't seroconvert until at least six weeks after they have been infected, so there is a lag time between exposure and a positive test result. A person who is infected on a Friday night and gets tested the following Monday, for example, will probably have a negative reading. But he or she will still be capable of infecting others. And even if the negative reading is accurate, three months of unprotected sex later it might not be. Often somebody who tells you they are "negative" is referring to a test they had five or six years ago. At the San Francisco AIDS

Foundation we recommend that everybody use condoms routinely unless they are in a strictly monogamous relationship and both parties have tested negative twice over a period of six months.

"Yeah, but . . . well, do you really think I could have gotten infected? I mean . . . he looked really healthy . . . we only did it two times . . . You don't think I'm in any danger, do you?"

How I desperately want to comfort them the way I comfort my little boy, to tell them it will be all right, that they should take a hot bath, listen to some soothing music, and forget about it all. But I can't do this. My voice sounds cruel and implacable to my own ears, like a prison warden locking cells and ignoring the pleas of the incarcerated. "You're definitely at risk. You should make an appointment to get tested."

I learn about sexual practices I never knew existed. Docking, for instance. I have to interrupt the young man who calls and ask him to explain this to me. His voice sounds blurry, unfocused. I form a swift image of him: tall, pug-nosed, white eyelashes. Grew up on a farm, used to fuck chickens. And, as he informs me, he has an uncircumcised penis. Which is why he is so popular at this sport called docking. You need one man who is "uncut" to stand in the center of the circle; one by one, the other men, who are circumcised, fit their penises into the "dock" created by pulling the center man's foreskin over their own member. To enhance the effect, cock rings are used to lock the two penises in place until one or both men come.

I feel mildly ill. I am quite fond of men in general but the more of their stories I hear, the more I realize that they are a very different sort of animal. I try hard not to be judgmental. We have been carefully trained not to question the erotic proclivities of our callers; instead, we draw their attention to the consequences of their acts, both for themselves and for their partners. Often this is a difficult line to tread. I feel much as I do when I explain to my little boy that he should not jump down the stairs three at a time, because there is the possibility that he *might* fall, although he never has yet: his response to my words of caution is always, "But, Mommy, I *like* to jump down the stairs."

"What made you call now?" I ask, more out of curiosity than a professional need to know. He's been docking for years.

"My mother died of cancer last week," he replies. "It got me to thinking."

"About—?"

"Oh, death and stuff. You know, deep stuff. My mom, she didn't know about me and other guys, but my dad did. He don't talk to me no more. So I don't have no family left, you know? I got all this deep shit in my mind. Thought about talking to this minister who read at my mom's funeral but then I figured it might be too much for him. So I called you guys."

I praise him for having the courage to call. The praise, I hope, will smooth the path ahead when I have to tell him the bad news about how much he is endangering himself.

Only rarely does someone call who actually has HIV, or who has been newly diagnosed. I get a call from a young African woman who has been married eight years, has three children and one on the way. She does not have an HIV diagnosis yet, but she's about to get one. Her husband has just confessed to her that for the last five years, he has known that he has been HIV positive. They have never once used a condom when having sex. She and her children have all been tested, and she is waiting for the results, which will be available in a few days. Her voice has a pleasant singsong accent. I imagine that there is something comfortable and whole about this woman, that every piece of

her fits into every other piece smoothly, nothing jars or pro-
trudes. And now, of course, she is about to be shattered.
Who she thought she was is not who she will be from now
on. She is fairly well-educated about transmission, about
the testing procedure. But her soft voice expresses bewil-
derment, apology, and flat denial.

"Excuse me, miss, but you do not really think I have
caught this? After all, my children are so young."

I am tongue-tied. She continues, her rhythmic voice dip-
ping into odd little valleys. "Surely not my babies, miss?
That cannot be true."

I force myself to ask, my pulse beating rapidly, whether
she has nursed her children.

"Of course, miss," she says, proudly. "Every single one
for a year."

She does not seem to understand that the virus can also
be transmitted from mother to child through breast milk.
Violating the principles of my job, I make a swift decision
to withhold this information from her. Instead, I tell her
about hope, the thing with feathers. I explain that until she
gets the test results back, she can be certain of nothing. In
the event that she does get bad news, however, she should
be aware that there have been many advances in drug therapy in the last few years. AIDS has become a manageable
illness. Well, for many people, anyhow. (My conscience
forces me to append this important qualification.) And, as
for children, they are living longer and longer. Some are
even going to college. I pelt her with referrals: to a pediatric
AIDS clinic, to a support group for families in her community, to a research and treatment hotline.

I detest myself. I sound like a flight attendant offering a
selection of menu choices.

The young woman rises above my pathetic good inten-
tions. "Well, miss, I thank you, but I am sure I will not need

these phone numbers. My children are too little. It is impossible for me to be sick. God would not allow it."

After I say goodbye to this woman, I put the phone on "Do Not Disturb" and take a break. I go to the bathroom and splash my sweaty face with water and reapply my make-up. Especially the lipstick.

I make it a rule not to disclose to any caller that I am HIV positive myself, no matter how much I am tempted. From experience, I've discovered that if I tell them, they invariably ask me, "How long are you going to live?" This would be a rude question under any circumstances, even if you were in the peak of health. But I'm not put off by the rudeness, and the question no longer frightens me. It merely embarrasses me, as if someone had asked me whether my pubic hair was turning gray. One's life span is such an intimate bodily topic: that question, actually, is the only one on this job that inspires me to prudery. I will talk about sex every which way to men, women, and all those in between, but I draw the line at inquiries into my personal longevity.

Most of my calls are routine. I spend about two-thirds of my time talking about oral sex, usually to men, debating its risks. The San Francisco AIDS Foundation takes an official position regarding oral sex: we are instructed to tell our callers that it is a "low risk" activity although not without risk altogether. In general, callers are disappointed by this response; everybody wants yes or no answers. It's only human nature. Gray areas, where doubt and ambiguity enter into play, are never popular, either in life or on the hotline. I participate in endless discussions about whether condoms are really necessary or not during this act. Men have all sorts of excuses for not using them, the most common being that they are "too large" to wear one comfortably. I gather that there are a disproportionate number of well-endowed men at loose in the state of California. But many are frightened about not using them, too, or about not insisting that their partner use one. If I detect this, I have a standard line I use: "I am hearing that you're anxious about this issue. And if you're at all fearful, even just a little bit, you should be using a condom." The locution "I am hearing" is pure hotline-ese. I keep thinking one of my callers is going to point out how ridiculous I sound, but nobody does. Sometimes when I get home I say to my little boy, "*I am hearing* that you want to eat fish sticks for supper." He laughs at me.

All this penis talk makes me think again about the end of sex. I remember when there used to be some mystique about the male organ, but here at the San Francisco AIDS Foundation we have so thoroughly deconstructed the penis that as a result I think of it as free-floating, totally divorced from the act of love-making. I suppose this is the way doctors learn to think of the entire human body: devoid of eroticism. I find it depressing. I know more about the anatomy of the penis than many men do. Sometimes, in a show-offy mood, I will talk to a man about his *meatus*. He clears his throat on the other end: "Pardon?" No, no, I think, this is all wrong, this textbook approach—give me back the penis the way it used to be, in all its mythological glory, its pomposity, its ferocity.

There is one sort of call I get at least once a shift, and it always begins like this: "Look, first of all, I want to say, I'm a married man, and I love my wife. But last night I . . . a) slept with a prostitute or b) let another man suck my dick." These men are certain that the weight of their guilt alone will be enough to press the virus into their bloodstream. They believe justice is swift, and that unless their confession is speedier, they are doomed. I am their confessor, handing out indulgences, dispensing stern words of comfort. After a little questioning, it usually turns out that the prostitute insisted on a condom. I point out that prostitutes often make much "safer" partners than the "average" woman you'd pick up in a bar. They're generally experienced professionals who know how to protect themselves, whereas the bar lady may use condoms only sporadically, if at all. The men who have had their first sexual experience with another man have a different kind of guilt to wrestle with. Most of them insist that they are straight and I take them at their word. Another thing I have learned during my year on the hotline is what a slippery business sexual identity can be. We have at least six categories of sexuality on our computer's demographic chart. "Men who have sex with men" is one I check off frequently on this sort of call, rather than "gay" or "bisexual."

Sometimes I hear a romance. The man who calls has a pleasant, halting voice, and I picture him as tall and a little burly, with wavy brown hair, perhaps in his early forties. He hails from a well-to-do suburb in the Bay Area. The sort of fellow who likes to dabble in carpentry on the weekends, building bird feeders and kitchen cabinets in his garage. He has big hands and feet. Happy, no money problems. I am not surprised when he tells me that he loves his wife and that they still have satisfying sex. Neither am I surprised when he tells me that for the last six months he has been having an affair with his next door neighbor—a man.

"You know, we didn't expect anything like this to happen. We've been living next door for five years and we're best friends. He's married too; our wives used to hang out together, but then his wife had a terrible accident, she's been paralyzed for over a year now. We golf together—he's a lot better than I am, he gives me a lot of pointers. He's always borrowing tools from me, cause they're building an addition to their house, lots of ramps and stuff for the wife.

Right around the time of the accident he began to talk to me a lot about how frightened he was, how confused he was feeling, like his whole life was ending. Sometimes he'd cry. I'd just listen to him. We're buddies—we help each other out, you know? Friends."

"Then one day . . . I don't even know how this happened . . . one day we were in his garage, I'd come over to loan him something, I forget what . . . it was raining out . . . we were just talking . . . and all of a sudden I look at his face and I get this kind of shock and I think, 'I love this man.' He sees me looking and he turns kind of red. Then he asks what I was thinking about. And I blurt it right out. I say, 'I love you, I'm attracted to you.' The rain is just pouring down outside so we're trapped in there telling each other the absolute truth. There's no way we can back out now. And he says, 'I'm glad you said that, because I think I'm falling in love with you too.'"

So far they have only indulged in oral sex, and always with a condom. They are both equally responsible; before they make their assignations, one or the other always thinks to make a trip to the drugstore first. The man asks me, shyly, for permission to "progress." By this he means to protected anal sex. I tell him that I cannot make up his mind for him. I praise him and his partner for behaving so responsibly. I remind him that he has his wife's safety to consider also. He struggles to explain himself, "It's hard to—to . . . It's not that I don't love my wife. I love her as much as ever. But I love this man too. I know that doesn't make much sense." I don't tell him but I think it makes perfect sense. I shock myself when I say, "If you and this man both want to go further, and if you use condoms religiously, then I'd say there's no reason why you shouldn't." I discover on this job that my strongest allegiance is to love—wherever it may surface. This man's tale has lifted my spirits so miraculously that I am willing to grant him any dispensation he wants. He thanks me profusely before he hangs up, assures me that I will be "in his prayers."

My shift on the hotline never ends without an encounter with one or several of our infamous "chronic callers." There is the classic voyeur, for example, who enjoys watching his wife have sex with other men. He cloaks his prurient interest in an all-too-legitimate concern about contracting HIV, a strategy that fools us at first. After we've heard from him many times we decide he is using us as a sounding board for his fantasies. He may or may not be masturbating; if he is, he's very quiet and controlled about it. Mostly, I think, he just wants to get the story right and he's willing to undertake endless revisions. It takes months to detect him. He is clever enough to change the details every time he calls, so that we will be forced to listen to him without hanging up, giving him the benefit of the doubt, just in case he really *is* someone different, someone desperately in need of our advice. My favorite call is the one where he claims his wife had breast implants that she could not afford; as payment, she gives the plastic surgeon a fancy fuck that involves all sorts of acrobatic feats, including one with a harness. Sometimes I find myself getting turned on by his soft voice and his descriptive passages; then I wonder at this man's power to break through all my defenses, to make a mockery at my attempt to be strictly clinical. He frightens me. After awhile I learn to recognize him and I hang up when he calls.

Nobody I know from my shift has actually spoken to the man who sleeps with his horse, but everybody claims to have known someone who has from another shift. He has always called just the day before or the hour before my shift begins. The man who sleeps with his horse is worried about getting HIV. He asks if he should be using a condom.

Then there's Ravi. Usually when I enter the room, one of the other volunteers will warn me, "Ravi's making the rounds today. He's already called two or three times." Ravi is a middle-aged Indian man who is committed to a mental hospital. Somehow he always manages to find a public phone to call us from, so he can't be one of the dangerous psychotic types who is locked up in a cell. I picture him as balding, with shiny skin that's always on the verge of breaking out in a sweat. He's very polite; he knows each one of us by name and he is overjoyed to hear our voices. He loves our society and thinks of us as his true friends.

"Hello, Ravi," I greet him.

"Why hello! Who is that? Is that Paula? Yes it is! I hope you are having so far a pleasant morning! Do you know, it is already eighty-nine degrees here? What temperature is it in San Francisco?"

"It's foggy."

"That's marvelous! So cool! I would like to be there at this moment!"

"Ravi, do you have a question about HIV today?"

"But I do! Yes, I do!"

He delivers an extremely well-structured question, obviously read straight from one of the pamphlets we distribute. This time it's about the possibility of contracting HIV through mutual masturbation. Ravi goes to great lengths not to repeat himself and thus to bore us: every call he pretends to have a different concern. His consideration touches me. He is too well-mannered to dispense with this small formality of acting the part of the "worried well" in order to have the pleasure of talking to us. He has figured out that we, for some mysterious reason, like to discuss this disease, and he obliges us. Actually, he humors us. I like him because he seems to regard HIV as a silly nursery tale that we all collectively cherish although we are way past the age of such belief—to Ravi, we are all grown-ups afraid of the boogey-man.

He barely listens to my answer; when I am finished, he bursts out, as if he has been impatiently holding himself in check. "Paula! Tell me, I must know, what do you think about President Clinton and these shenanigans with China?"

"I don't know. I haven't been thinking much about it, I guess."

"Why, I think of it constantly! I study the question very seriously. I read everything, do you know? Here is what I read: *U.S. News and World Report, USA Today, Newsweek, Time,* the *New York Times, People Magazine,* the *San Francisco Chronicle, Vogue, Entertainment Weekly.* Oh, also, the *Wall Street Journal.* I have read all of those just this morning."

"You've been busy, Ravi."

"Oh, I like to keep informed. I learn so many interesting things, you can't imagine! The world is a quite fascinating place, Paula."

"You're telling me."

"I think you should read more."

"I should."

We chat a bit longer; he chides me, gently, for my ignorance regarding the China question and advises me to subscribe to more newspapers. Then I notice my supervisor making slicing gestures across his neck.

"Well, Ravi, have I answered your question about HIV?"

"Oh yes, in a most lucid manner! I am forever grateful."

"Then I'll have to say goodbye. I have another call on hold."

"But of course. Delightful talking to you, as usual! Perhaps the weather will warm up for you and it will cool down for me, and then all of life will be perfect, will it not?"

"Let's hope so, Ravi."

"Goodbye, then!"

"Goodbye."

And so it goes. Four hours straight I put my finger in the dike to hold back the huge wave of fear and terror and insanity threatening to overwhelm the human race. Fondly, I imagine that thousands of men are now using condoms correctly because of my advice. ("Never use an oil-based lubricant. Roll out the air bubbles. And for God's sake check the expiration date.") That thousands of women will now buy condoms themselves and insist that their partners use them. That the "worried well" will start dating again. That HIV, the *bête noire* of my own life too, has suffered a severe blow to its self-esteem, and that from now on it will realize that humanity and love and sex are not mere fodder for its hellish appetite. All these airy fantasies sustain me for the week between my shifts.

Chapter Seven

Mothers on Capitol Hill

At the age of thirty-nine, on the brink of middle age, I set out to save the world. I am an activist. Tentatively I mouth these words, and by the third or fourth time I have spoken this sentence, it begins to seem credible. Could I be an activist? *Am* I an activist? Yes, I am. I *am* an activist. Well, at least for the time being, anyhow.

I have good reason to doubt myself, because for most of my life I have been indifferent to world affairs. It is only in the last few years that I have developed a political conscience. Once, in graduate school, I got dragged into a march against apartheid, but it was only because I was on my way to the library and the marchers happened to cross my path and one of them was my advisor, who pulled me in, and I felt for the sake of my academic career I couldn't refuse. Even voting, I am ashamed to say, was a duty I performed only sporadically, at best. I voted in national elections, but not local ones; I could not muster enough interest in most issues to learn about them.

Now here I am, three and a half years after a diagnosis that left me scrambling to rehabilitate my personality, getting turned on by what people can achieve with their voices, their wills. People could achieve things with their writing, but it was a slower process. I want to be heard, and for once I have something to say that other people might be interested in hearing, and this is a compelling motivation in itself, never mind the political one. So in March of the year 2000 I travel to Washington, D.C. to participate in an annual lobbying event staged by the National Association of People With AIDS (NAPWA) called AIDSWATCH. Our goal is to convince members of Congress to vote in favor of renewal of the Ryan White CARE Act, a federally funded but state-allocated program that provides many invaluable social and medical services for people with AIDS. It includes a separate title providing an umbrella of services for women and children. If the CARE Act is not renewed, and at funding levels significantly above what has originally been allocated, many people with HIV/AIDS will be left out in the cold.

I am traveling with Felicia Court. Felicia is leading a troupe of women to Washington and guiding us through the intricacies of the legislative process. She will be my Virgil. Felicia's eldest daughter was diagnosed with AIDS in 1987 and died in 1992 and Felicia, a lifelong activist with roots in the civil rights era, suddenly found herself enlisted in a new cause. She is the founder of a grassroots advocacy group made up of mothers of children who have HIV/AIDS, or mothers who are living with HIV/AIDS themselves. Many advocacy groups are converging in Washington from all over the country for the AIDSWATCH event, and I am grateful to be counted among Felicia's number.

Felicia is the most beautiful sixty-four-year-old woman I have ever seen. I can't stop looking at her face, at its various perfections: the forty-carat nose, the lapidary cheekbones. She has a disarming smile, all white teeth and radiance. Her eyes are disturbing—they're huge, deep-set, honey amber. And they're a paradox—such a warm Mediterranean color, and yet what a cold, Arctic light they shed. She glitters, like the blade of a sword in winter sunlight.

Felicia wears her straight, silvery-white hair upswept in an elegant French twist, with bangs falling to her eyebrows. I never see her wear her hair any other way, and her style seems as much a statement of character as it is an indicator of vanity; she maintains, in all venues, from boardroom to soup kitchen, an aura of determined glamour, as if, by God, life can hand her what it will, but her beauty is her shield, and it shall not be pierced.

Her vanity has been an asset to her in the legislative corridors of San Francisco's City Hall, Sacramento's assemblies, and Capitol Hill in Washington, D.C., where she has spent many days of her life. Politicians, especially men, let down their guard with her. She tells a terrific story about a visit with a coalition of concerned citizens to then Governor Pete Wilson of California, a crafty man whose tactical approach to lobbyists and earnest citizens' coalitions consisted of talking so much and with such dry fluency that by the end of these meetings (strictly limited to fifteen minutes) his was the only voice that was ever heard. A political advisor suggested that he might want to let a constituent say a word or two. Governor Wilson grudgingly admitted the wisdom of this advice. In the meeting which Felicia attended his eyes swept over the group of ten, and were arrested by Felicia's face. What indictments could come from such a flawless mouth? He nodded and encouraged her to speak. And she proceeded to tell him exactly what she thought of his policies regarding immigration and the proposition just now being drafted that would deny health care to illegal aliens.

Although Felicia did not swear at Governor Wilson, in her private, non-official encounters, she has a truly foul mouth. "I learned how to say 'fuck' for the first time when my daughter was sick," she says. Then laughs: "And I've been saying it ever since!"

It's because people are always fucking up that Felicia is in this business. You have to be on the alert for the fuck-ups: you have to be a critic on a gargantuan scale, tackling lily-livered governments and blighted legislation and fossilized school districts. Mediocrity is her archenemy. She can't open her mouth without uttering a complaint—"Excuse me, sir, I have to tell you, you need to buy new shocks for this cab! I'm going to have to sue you for kidney damage!" In a world that accommodates AIDS, is it any wonder Felicia howls?

In the van we've managed to coerce into driving us from the airport in Baltimore to our hotel in D.C. for only ten dollars a head (the driver is beguiled by Felicia's flirting, the press of female bodies surrounding him, our siren's voices, our sheer neediness), we have a discussion about faith. Felicia makes some mention of nuns in her girlhood. "Are you a practicing Catholic?" I ask her. She replies, "Oh, honey, I practiced it so hard I got it right and I don't need to practice anymore." Now she spends most of her days in a Lutheran church, where she is the director of a program that provides services for homeless people with HIV. Twice a month she throws elegant banquets for the hapless infected. (I imagine her bitching at the caterers.) The pastor is a great friend of hers, a great supporter of her program and of people with HIV in general. Felicia reveres him. He is one of the few people I have ever heard her speak of without irony.

Felicia is still very much a Catholic, I think, in spite of her protestations, and in spite of her affiliation with a Lutheran church. I think of Graham Greene and his eloquent wrestling with faith, his absolute determination to subdue it and his ultimate, tortured surrender, in novel after novel. And I think, what a pity Graham Greene is not around to write a novel about Felicia.

Our first full day in Washington, NAPWA holds an orientation and training seminar, and that evening at dinner Felicia denounces their lack of foresight and planning. Indeed, she has much to complain about. Packets of vital information about the representatives' voting records on key issues are missing because the "copy machine was broken." Breakfast and bottled water—crucial for people with suppressed immune systems in a city that has a notoriously contaminated water supply—which NAPWA had promised to provide never materialize. "Let me tell you, honey, I honed my ass in corporate America," says Felicia. "And if I'd been responsible for planning a conference that turned out like this one, I wouldn't have a job the next morning." She blames, in particular, NAPWA's new acting director. "That goddamned dyke or *whatever* it is, I have a problem with her. She's a control freak. We offered to help her organize this event—the San Francisco AIDS Foundation was willing to pitch in too—but she wasn't having any of it." Actually the director is not a dyke but a person in transition from womanhood to manhood: a transsexual. He's hefty, with large breasts and hips that unfortunately cannot be disguised by clothing, and one is left with a sense of gender adrift, unspecified. Felicia has no patience with him. "She has a goddamned chip on her shoulder the size of a boulder. Let me tell you, she wasn't glad to see *me* here with my big mouth. You know what it is she doesn't like the most? The fact that I'm all woman, baby, and she can't manage to be one thing or another."

By morning, Felicia's venomous mood is dispelled. She shows up for our first day of lobbying with a serene smile, looking like a million bucks in black slacks, a black and gray striped turtleneck sweater, and dynamite silver jewelry. Maureen, an attorney who works for an organization that gives free legal advice to people with AIDS, compliments her. Maureen is a pleasant-looking, unadorned female, who is earnest, chipper, optimistic, and kind—everything that Felicia is not. Felicia waves her hand. "Oh, honey, it's all an illusion. I feel like hell. I'm getting too old for this. Old ladies like me should be sitting on a beach in Hawaii, sipping Mai-tais. Wouldn't that be the life?"

In all my trips to Washington, I have never visited Capitol Hill—with the possible exception of a class trip in the eighth grade, although I remember little about that except giggling in my hotel room and trying to sneak a peek at some boys in the room across the way. Most of my visits, I gravitate toward the National Gallery and the Hirshhorn, ignoring the government. But here I am, all dressed up in a conservative gray suit (not my style) and sensible shoes, ready for an assault on the legislative body. I am impressed by the solid whiteness of the Capitol itself and the contrasting delicacy of the lacy pink cherry blossoms and the rows of stately pink tulips. How beautiful it is, the epicenter of the free world. The two buildings that encompass the House of Representatives are rather more prosaic: except for a few showy hallways with marble floors and doorways draped with flags in the old sections of the buildings, most of the corridors remind me of my elementary school. The linoleum is scuffed, there are janitors mopping up, old-fashioned wooden phone booths. I had expected—what—something more Louis the Sixteenth perhaps? Pages with white wigs to usher us into the inner sanctum?

We have been divided into groups of five to seven, and we have fifteen minutes to tell our stories and make our requests. Maureen, the attorney, preps us: "Be sure to get a commitment out of them. That's the important thing.

They're all going to be polite, nobody's going to be hostile to a group of people with HIV. But don't be sucked in by that; just because they've listened to you doesn't mean they're going to give us what we want."

Felicia interjects, "Boo-hoo-hoo, more people with AIDS, that's what they're really thinking. They've seen us coming and going. They think, just tell them what they want to hear and get rid of them."

"Well, it's not as bad as all that, Felicia," says Maureen. "These people have a conscience, it's just that they have a lot of other things on their agendas."

"*We're* their fucking conscience," says Felicia. "Don't you forget that, ladies. We make them wake up and smell the shit. And speaking of ladies—I take it back, they haven't seen a lot of us coming and going. They need to open their eyes and take a good look at us."

And I suddenly remember why I'm here: I'm white, I'm middle-class, I'm well-educated, and I look like Senator So-and-So's niece or daughter or sister-in-law. I've been chosen for my shock value. Our biggest enemy, what we've really come to fight, is the attitude that AIDS is a disease that happens to *other* people. Our second biggest enemy is the mistaken belief that the disease no longer poses a significant threat: that it's a sort of low-simmer illness, something that you can safely leave on the back burner while you attend to other things.

Maureen gives us a few last-minute tips on how to close a deal; Felicia draws her rookies together in a huddle for a pep talk. All the groups will have a facilitator, an experienced lobbyist who will direct the meeting and make sure everything that needs to be said gets said. Some of the facilitators are women but some are gay men. In particular, two natty dudes from the policy department of the San Francisco AIDS Foundation, the sort of men straight women find themselves falling in love with even though they know better. They look terrific in their well-cut suits, the trousers breaking just so. One has a shaved head and broad shoulders and a winning smile; the other is elfin, with lovely fair skin and clever slanting eyes. Both of them stand poised to perform, actors strutting in the wings before curtain time.

Felicia glances at these men suspiciously and whispers to us, "Those guys are smooth, they've been doing this for years. Don't let them steamroll you. Yes, it's true, they began this fight and it's because of them that we've made such enormous progress. We couldn't have done it without them. But they're not the only voices anymore, and they need to know that. You just go right ahead and say what you need to in your own voice. If I hear one of those candy-asses isn't letting you talk, they'll have me to answer to."

The elfin one pricks up his ears, laughs nervously. "What are you doing over there, Felicia?"

"Oh, just girl talk," she replies, eyes sparking dangerously.

I am ready to begin. But here is my old fear of closed doors, the anxiety about when to knock, and when to enter. Why would they want us to come in, anyhow, won't we be disturbing them? They're busy *governing*, for God's sake, aren't they? But I soon learn that it is our business to walk in. This is America, we can walk in and out with our demands and grievances. If our legislators are not accessible to their constituents, they will lose their jobs. I think to myself, what a job, having to see people and talk to them all the time. Privacy is unheard of, frowned upon. Of all the professions, a politician's is the most foreign to my own nature.

I discover that it is rare to actually meet with your congressperson. Instead, you meet with his or her staff. I attend nine meetings in the two days of lobbying and I never speak to my elected official. (Nancy Pelosi, my representative from San Francisco, who has been instrumental in supporting

AIDS causes, pokes her head in the door of our meeting with her legislative analyst to say hello on the way to a congressional hearing—she has the merry, insouciant air of a popular girl who gets invited to too many parties.) Maureen assures us that this is perfectly normal and that staff are almost as powerful as their bosses; they have the ear of the congressperson, and make recommendations regarding many important bills and propositions. But to me, they look suspiciously young. I am almost old enough to be their mother. (Felicia grumbles, "How old was that last kid we saw? Thirteen? My granddaughter is eighteen and she could eat him for breakfast.") I never see anyone fifty or older in Washington. I get the feeling the free world is being run by youngsters. In one office, all the available space is crowded with baby paraphernalia—a swing, a stroller, bottles and diapers. The legislative analyst appears with a ten-month-old baby in her arms; there are dark smudges under her eyes and she listens to our virtuous demands with a distracted air. At another visit the staffperson is a young Republican; he wears the requisite navy blazer with gold buttons. When one woman in our party addresses the pressing need for more global aid, especially for the African countries hard hit by the disease, he responds wearily, "Of course, the real solution is to enable these countries to become self-sufficient financially . . . Instead of throwing money at them, we feel that our best efforts toward combating this disease will be to support their economy with legislation that encourages free trade . . ."

The youth and, in general, the friendliness and encouragement of these staffers has a beneficial effect: it dispels my nervousness. I look them right in the eye and give them my three-minute spiel: my diagnosis in the midst of nursing my child; my life saved at an advanced stage of the disease due to powerful drugs which would not have existed without the NIH, and without the funding allocated to the NIH; the many services that have helped improve the quality of my life. I try to forget that I am really just a glorified beggar dressed up in a suit—I might as well be holding out my hand palm up—and with chin raised, I ask them if they will support renewal of the CARE act along with other important legislative and budgetary requests we are making. And would they, could they, give me an answer about how they will vote? Before I leave the room? As I speak I begin to feel curiously divided from myself—my story is a genuinely sad one, and I can tell from the expressions on the faces of my listeners that I have delivered it convincingly, and yet after many tellings I no longer feel any emotional connection to it. The absence of self-pity is probably a healthy thing. Still, I am selling myself, making a show of my deepest and most personal tragedy, and yet, how else is it to be done? As my life story morphs into a story *about* my story (and I revise as I go along, sharpening a detail here, omitting a detail there), I begin to understand that there is an element of performance in even the noblest of human endeavors. And there's a way, too, of balancing honesty with craft. Maybe speechifying is not so different from writing, after all.

I learn, gradually, of all the ways Felicia's life has fallen apart, of all the fuck-ups. There have been two failed marriages, major debts, her granddaughter's bouts with clinical depression, her other children's hostility to her in the face of her utter consecration to their stricken sister. The granddaughter will be off to college soon in another state; the other children have scattered, leaving their self-motivated and self-sufficient mother to her own devices.

I feel a strong kinship with Felicia. I'm also a proud survivor of my own fuck-ups.

We have several meetings together. With a contemptuous glance at the latest baby-faced analyst, she draws three photographs out of her purse and throws them on the table before her. Gingerly, the analyst picks them up. Felicia states, "That's my daughter. She died of AIDS eight years ago. And that's my granddaughter, her daughter, whom I'm raising on my own . . ." Her tone implies: "I don't give a damn who you are or how you judge me. These lives I'm putting before you mean more than yours will ever mean. If you have any sense, you'll vote the way we tell you to."

Afterward, I ask to see the photographs. One is of her daughter sitting at a table, chin in hand: she is cute, petite, with Felicia's huge brown eyes. In another, she is bedridden, suffering from partial paralysis and dementia, Felicia explains, but she has mustered a crooked smile for a cake on the night table—it's a celebration of her thirty-fourth birthday, which as it turns out is her last. The last photo is of a strapping blond teenager caught in a moment of joy—standing on her toes, arms flung above her head.

Felicia is wry about this girl. "That little hussy is so spoiled. And guess who's responsible? This old grandma has to get up every morning at the crack of dawn and drive her to school. I mean, God forbid she should have to take the bus. That girl's feet have not touched public transportation since she was five years old." On the last day of our trip, she drags me along on a search for a Victoria's Secret store. "Last time I went to Washington I didn't know what to bring her back so I got her eight pairs of thong panties. She thought I was the best grandma in the entire world."

As we are scurrying down a corridor on our way from one meeting to another, I ask Felicia what has become of her granddaughter's father.

"Oh, honey, my daughter was a drug addict. She was extremely promiscuous; God only knows who the father was.

I mean, she was married to this guy and he may have been the father. Hell, he wanted custody of Beth after Jeannine divorced him and came to live with me, after she learned she was sick, see. So maybe he was the dad. Beth was five years old at the time her mom came back to me. Jeannine and I hadn't spoken for six years."

Suddenly she grasps my arm and the arm of the woman on the other side of her. Her voice catches; her cold amber eyes are filled with tears.

Maureen, who is ahead of us, turns around nervously. "Oh, Felicia, don't. No. You promised. Not now . . ."

But Felicia continues. "Six years! She didn't want to have anything to do with me. But in the end we were reconciled. I nursed her until the last minute. I did it myself, with just a little outside help. I held her in my arms when she died."

Maureen shakes her head, clicks her teeth, appeals to me. "Don't let her. She *promised* me . . ."

In a taxi from the Senate building back to our hotel in Foggy Bottom, Felicia informs me that her second husband owned a department store that she helped manage. For a while they were wealthy, hobnobbing with some of the important figures in California retail. Then there were debts, bankruptcy. Felicia landed on her feet, opened up a highly successful boutique on Union Street in San Francisco. But when her daughter returned to live with her, and Felicia devoted her life to nursing her and caring for the daughter's small child, she was forced to sell her business, at a significant loss. What money was left over fed the legal costs of an epic custody battle.

We are taking a break in the room NAPWA has provided for AIDSWATCH participants, sipping orange sodas and watching the rain outside the window. "When I first saw that kid, she was malnourished. She was five years old and looked like a three year old. They weren't giving her enough to eat, do you understand? And one of the guys my daughter was fucking, maybe it was the one who was masquerading as Beth's dad, who knows, had been poking her with his dick. I kid you not. A little creature like that. There was nothing I could do but go to court. And I was up against that father and his wealthy Marin County family. To this day my name is famous in the San Francisco courts. I didn't have one goddamned dime to my name when it was over. But it was worth it, because I saved her life."

As we stand in line to board a plane that will take us home, Felicia, speaking half over her shoulder, sums up her maternal career for me: "If you asked my two sons what they thought of me as a mother and then if you asked my daughters, you'd get completely different stories. The boys thought I was okay. But the girls. I was beautiful, intelligent, and successful, and they hated me for that."

On the evening before our departure, Felicia gathers all the women she has shepherded to Washington in her hotel room for a debriefing. She intends this to be a serious discussion of what we have accomplished and what we still need to accomplish in the future, but the discussion degenerates into a voicing of complaints. We have all been allotted a sum of money for this trip and most of us feel the amount has been generous. Several of the women, however, have spent all their money and have nothing left to get them from the airport to their homes. One woman has been begging money from a few other women in the group, myself included. We suspect she may be an alcoholic and has been tippling the expensive bottles of liquor found in the hotel room refrigerators. Felicia patiently explains how difficult it was to scrape together the funds, from donations and small grants, to pay for this trip, and how important it is to learn how to manage our money. At this, one of the women bristles: she accuses Felicia of not understanding the difficulties of their lives, the struggle to live on disability and general assistance payments when you have six kids, the unforeseen emergencies that drain cash. "How dare you tell me I don't know how to manage money!" she shouts. Another woman, unable to tolerate the arguing, leaves the room. Two others begin to whisper together. Our solidarity is threatened; something must be done.

It's true Felicia has been condescending. Condescension comes so naturally to her, she forgets how it affects others. And, indeed, she looks queenly, sitting with her back held so straight, her hair upswept and her pink sweater set adorned with a string of faux pearls. Anybody could be enraged by her at this moment: all that super-efficiency, that brittle correctness of manner. Yet I know Felicia is not about to apologize to anybody—after all, aside from choosing the wrong tone of voice, she hasn't been guilty of any error. I am curious as to how she will handle the situation; if I were in her position, I would certainly be red-faced and groveling by now.

She says, "Honey, I may have started out life with something in my pocket but now I'm just an old lady looking forward to my social security payments. Every extra penny I make is going straight to my granddaughter's tuition. Her so-called father owes me fifty thousand dollars in child support, but do you think there's a chance in hell I'm ever going to see any of that? I don't *think* so." Her upper lip begins to quiver, and she waves her right hand in the air. Somebody puts a tissue in it. "When my daughter was lying there sick and half paralyzed, I had to work two part-time jobs to keep the wolf from the door—I couldn't work full-time during the day because I was taking care of Jeannine, so I worked every evening from 6 to 10 P.M. waitressing and all day on weekends as a saleswoman at Macy's. Jeannine's siblings or friends of mine took turns watching

Jeannine and Beth while I was gone. I was working all day long, seven days a week, from the moment I put my feet out of bed in the morning till the moment I crawled into bed again way past midnight. And then I was up lots of nights taking care of Jeannine too. So don't anyone, *anyone* ever tell me I don't know the meaning of hard work and struggle."

There is silence; the woman who spoke up looks at her lap, chastened. Eyes peeking above a veil of tissue covering the lower half of her face, Felicia surveys her flock. Now she has us where she wants us; now she can get back to business. All of the above story is true, of course. But if it had not been delivered with such consummate skill, it might not be so convincing.

Felicia understands, from years of dealing with politicians, that the world is not so much about good guys and bad guys; it's all about whose version of events gains the upper hand. It's not enough to cleave to your principles or stake out your position on the moral high ground; if you want your story told, then you'd better damn well know how to package it, sell it, and shout it out loud.

Back in San Francisco, in the busy airport, Felicia says goodbye to me, then remarks, with a firm nod, "Our paths will cross again." I am thrilled to hear it.

Chapter Eight

Letter to Benjamin

Dear Benjamin,

How could you ever know how many hours I spend trying to imagine what your face will look like when you are an adult? Now you are two, and your dear face is a fundamental fact of my universe. Like all the best and truest faces, it is idiosyncratic: I have already identified the faint puckering under the eyes, the two crescent-moons that indented my own childish face and are deeply imprinted on my mature one. That indentation under the eyes is an inherited trait, and it mars your perfect babyness in a happy, humanizing fashion. Because of those lines you will never be able to advertise children's clothes in a catalogue or perform silly tricks on television. On my own face, as a child, these lines often made me look sleep-deprived, or, worse, sickly, although neither was usually true. On your face they give the same impression of unnatural weariness, as if you have been up all night in your crib philosophizing. As an adult the lines aged me by several years and gave me a look of wisdom—although there was no more foundation in reality for this wisdom than there was for my appearance of sickliness as a child. I suppose I decided that since I could not rid myself of what I considered to be a flaw, I would turn it to my advantage. But since one's face is one's destiny, perhaps I finally did grow into the solemnity I had been merely aping in my youth. The lines affected my idea of who I was, after all, and every time I looked in the mirror (sometimes a hundred times a day as a teenager!) this idea was reinforced. How will the lines appear on your adult face, and to what will you ascribe them, to what use will you put them, and all your other features?

Your face has other flaws and surprises. For one thing, your complexion is not pretty. You are very fair—a legacy from your Polish-Jewish grandmother?—but it is not that lovely poetic pallor of the Irish, which must be set off by dark hair to be truly appreciated. My own skin has some olive. You have little color at all in your skin, no pink, except when you are sleeping and your cheeks are flushed. To give your complexion credit, it is not sallow either. It is a serviceable skin, that is all. I have even noticed a few blackheads on your cheeks—a sign of a passionate nature? Now I slather lotion on your face when we are out in the sun, but you will have to mind this for yourself when you are older—your father inclines to freckles and moles and has had a bout with melanoma. Your skin poses dangers and is, unfortunately, unfashionable.

Your eyes are a dark blue, inherited from your father, but otherwise unremarkable. The eyebrows show promise— they are still only faintly etched, since you are fair, but I can already see the devilish peaks that so attracted me in your father's face. The only question is what color they will become, and whether they will turn bushy like his or remain fine-lined. When you throw your whole face into a grin, your eyebrows stretch high on your forehead in a ridiculous but lovable way and then I remember that nobody grins like this as an adult: we keep our grins in check, and we soon learn which distortions of our features are acceptable, which not.

Your nose is still debatable: some think it will be long and straight like your maternal grandmother's, others argue that it will become a small, neatly formed structure, like your father's. Certainly both arguments have merit at this point. Again, when you smile, your nose is distorted, flattened and fattened at the flanks, not always attractively. In photographs it tends to be more pronounced and appears bigger than it is, which lends fuel to the large-nosed camp. It is the same with your mouth, a subject of endless discussions—will your lips be full, like mine and like my own father's—or will they be thin, like your father's? I secretly hope for fullness, ascribing this characteristic to a more generous nature, a more loving heart, a more sensual, emotional, and artistic temperament—although I know these are clichés which have little basis in reality, that full-lipped people can also turn out to be mean-spirited and narrow-minded. I search your face at all angles—profile, full-face, three-quarters, and upside down, and in all activities—sleeping, playing, yawning, sucking, laughing, eating. Sometimes in all these shifting images I catch sight for a moment of the Peterson underlip—and I cry out in glee and point it out to whoever may be standing by. And in another instant your expression changes and I lose my vision, I see only a generic mouth, without any distinguishing characteristics.

As to your chin, your cheekbones, your forehead—who knows? These things remain to be seen. Your light-brown (not truly blond, as flattery will have it) curly hair should not even be mentioned—it is considered your hallmark right now, by people who do not know you so well as I do. In my mind, referring to you as "the little boy with curly blond hair" is a reduction that does you, and all that you are, an injustice. And the hair will change, of course—it will get darker, coarser, thinner, experience tells us. At two your mutability is infinite. I like to think that I would always recognize you, even if I were to leave now and not see you again until thirty years later—but I am frightened, because I cannot concretely imagine your face as an adult. Sometimes it seems to me it will look one way, sometimes another. I cannot fix upon one version. Not even looking at your father's face will help, because, although you resemble him strongly, you do not resemble him completely.

I love your face more than anybody's in the world. I cannot quite accept the fact that I may not be permitted to see it through its infinite refinements, retrenchments, regroupings. A face at six, at ten, at fifteen, at twenty-two, at thirty-seven, at forty-two—these are all important faces. To a mother, one cannot take precedence over another, although the possessor of the face may favor one version for reasons of vanity or social acceptance. I give thanks every day that I have been graced by your two-year-old face, but I am greedy—I want to see *all* your faces, straight on through the progression of time. After all, I have scanned several other dear faces through the decades—the faces of my two parents, the faces of my closest friends. To think that *your* face, the most important in the world—that this face may be denied to me. I feel cheated on a grand scale. You should know that I have a serious illness and that my use of the phrase "the progression of time" is an act of daring for me.

You may wonder why I dwell so exclusively on your face, why I neglect to mention your character or the future milestones of your life. The answer is that of course I wonder about much more than your appearance—like all mothers, I muse about where you will go to school, what sort of work you will do, who you will marry (or not marry), the children you may or may not have, where you will live and what, finally, you will choose to love in this life. I have all sorts of fond ideas about how I would like you to conduct yourself, what precepts I would like you to live by, what to reject and what to embrace. Someday I will make a list of them for you, because you might find them interesting and maybe even instructive. But the truth is that I don't spend so much time wondering how your character will evolve because from the moment you were born I had a handle on it—that's nothing unusual for a mother.

People assure me that your relentless crying had something to do with colic, but I think otherwise—I am convinced that it was not indigestion, but sheer indignation at the fact that you could not move as you pleased, see and do what you pleased, because you were trapped in a body that you did not know how to operate yet, and you found that unconscionable. As well you should have—there's nothing picturesque about helpless infancy. Having been ill, I often imagine how it would feel to be completely dependent on another human being for all my needs, to lie flat on my back all day and surrender my body to somebody else's manipulations. And not always skillful or insightful manipulations either—mostly basic ones, probably. I like to believe that when my time comes I will display the same ruthlessness, that I will take you as my example and let the world know how purely outraged I am at the condition I find myself in. And if no one listens, why, I'll just scream louder and longer, until *something* is done, and I will not suffer fools gladly during this time of dire need, and I will not waste any precious energy wondering whether I am interrupting someone's dinner or dragging someone away from the last chapter of a book. Under *no* circumstances do I want an odor of sanctity lingering near my corpse: I do not want anybody to say, "She was such a good patient; she always thought of other people, even when she was suffering the most." What nonsense. It's *you* I want to emulate. You with your strung-out nervous system, your flailing fists and arched back, your utterly uncompromising commitment to escape from the constraints nature has so unfairly placed upon you.

So you see that you were no whimperer, no bleater. You were a wailer, an extremist. You were clear about what you wanted from life, even at six days old. *Especially* at six days old. You would start with the breast but you refused to be put to bed directly after it; you insisted upon having a look around first, seeing what else was out there. Now that you are walking for yourself—your mood improved after this long-awaited event—you are not satisfied with conventionally delineated boundaries. At the playground, you refuse to hang out in the sandy area with the swings and slides— you run straight off to where the big kids are playing basketball, right up to the gate. You are fond of lurking near the perimeters.

I was not nearly so adventurous myself as a child. I remember that I was shy of knocking on doors I had never opened before (or which had not been first opened for me by an adult), and always faced a horrible awkwardness when deciding whether to open or not to open after the knock. (What if I could not hear someone say "come in?" What if they did not really say "come in" but I thought they did? What if there was no one there and I was caught trespassing?) I was familiar with my neighborhood up to a certain point, but no farther; the rest was fuzzy. This fuzziness began toward the middle of my block and became more pronounced at the far end. There were certain parts of houses—even familiar houses—I didn't explore, not because they were frightening or forbidding, but because my private taboos prevented me. In the house I lived in as a child for ten years, I never once entered a small room just beyond the main basement—a musty, low-ceilinged storage area with peeling plaster and a narrow window that looked out onto a neglected patch of grass near our front steps. I never knew what we stored there, and I liked it that way. I liked restrictions; I created them myself if they didn't exist. Why did I do this? Fear, partially, but also, probably, as a stimulant to imagination. Instinct informed me that it would be much more gratifying to imagine that basement room as a gateway to an alien galaxy from which, if I entered, I could never return, than to walk into it and discover boxes full of old photograph albums, cracked tea sets, and yellowing linen napkins. As you can see, I possessed a lot of Byzantine notions as a kid, although I was only half-conscious of them. You, however, would immediately penetrate and conquer that back room, subjugate it to your own uses.

I realize as I am writing this that while I can make a reasonable claim to understand something about your character, I am not at all certain that you have any conscious understanding of who I am. We have known each other now for two and a half years, but in many ways I have the advantage in this relationship—I view everything from an adult perspective, from the standpoint of experience, and with an adult's fluid sense of time, which can move backwards and forwards, sliding from past to future to present again with the greatest of ease. Much has been written lauding the ability of children to live wholly in the present tense. Many adults, facing crises and uncertainties in their lives, or simply wishing to live in a more happy fashion, have been counseled to strive to live as children do, for the moment and in the moment. But I am not always sure that this is such wise advice—I am fond of introspection and reflection and interpretation and analysis, all those adult qualities. I have a sense of history that you do not. If someone I loved dearly were to die now, I would remember this person for the rest of my born days. I would remember the first time we ever saw each other, and the last. I would replay again and again the many hours we spent together—meals we shared, jokes, books we'd read in common, walks we'd taken. I would be able to see my friend's face any time I pleased; all I would have to do is close my eyes in order to summon it forth. I would catalogue all my friend's accomplishments, and, having loved this person, I would probably embellish these accomplishments until with the passage of time they had become monumental achievements. All this and more I would do for someone I loved.

But will you be able to do these things for me?

The answer is no. Not because you don't love me—it's clear that you do love me. I appear to be the sun around which you slavishly orbit. I must say that no one I've known has ever loved me in this particular way before. It's almost embarrassing, because it's clear to me that I am no sun. But I go on pretending to be the sun, because that's what's best for you right now.

Insufficient love is not the problem. What it comes down to is this: you are simply too young. You are still a primitive, a demi-savage; if you stretch you can just manage to see over the rim of the present moment, and you are incapable of appreciating any of the subtle pleasures of delayed gratification. You are pre-literate. It will still be several years before you can read this letter and maybe several more years before you can understand it. So how can I expect you to keep me alive in your consciousness, when consciousness has barely dawned for you? When I first learned of my illness, I wished to die instantaneously, in order to spare you the sorrow of having to lose a mother who had come into focus for you as a human being—I reasoned that if you did not yet know me, then your loss would not be as severe. Now I am much more selfish; I pray every morning that I will be able to live long enough so that you will remember me forever, no matter how much suffering you have to undergo first. I have changed my mind: now I believe that, after all, it would *not* be better for you never to have known me. Your suffering might be more prolonged in that scenario; in fact, it might last forever. You might always be looking for me—whether consciously or unconsciously—and not being able to find me could make you miserable. You might feel abandoned; that is one of my worst fears. If I live long enough to come into focus for you as a human being, you will at least have the comfort of understanding that I did not leave you intentionally.

In the first wild weeks of grief after my diagnosis, I consulted several people traditionally deemed capable of dispensing comfort to someone in my situation. The first was a rabbi who told me that she herself had lost her father when she was a year old, and that while she didn't remember him, she had always sensed him as a "presence" in her life. The second was a psychiatrist who assured me that the foundations of a child's character are formed in the first few years of life, that their ability to love and be loved depends on what they learn in these years. Essentially, she was telling me not to worry, because although I was going to die, I had already given enough to you, I had done my part. What a relief! As you can imagine, I gleaned scant comfort from either person's advice. The rabbi and the psychiatrist were both professionals who offered me what their training and experience counseled them would be most useful and truthful. Well, I despised their professionalism.

Who wants to be a "presence?" And what mother could possibly be satisfied with hearing that two years with her child will be sufficient? I have a friend with three children—the youngest exactly your age—who was diagnosed

with multiple sclerosis at about the same time I was diagnosed with AIDS. She told me, "I can't very well die now,
because what use would I be to anybody six feet underground?" I think of this pragmatic Scots woman whenever
I fall into the trap of seeing my fate as other people, including the rabbi and the psychiatrist, must see it—as something tragic, inexorable, incontestable.

So, you see, I am determined that you *shall* know me.
That is probably the real reason I am writing you this letter,
because I want to present myself to you, as clearly as I can,
and while I am still able to. The task I set myself may be impossible, but I am determined not to cave in beneath doubts
and difficulties. I have faith that you can know me. Even if I
fall short of knowing myself, I feel sure that you will be able
to make up for my deficiencies. You will have to do some
work too—fill in the gaps, exercise your imagination, project yourself back in time. Readers and writers both have
their allotted tasks. But, a reader who is the progeny of the
writer has a certain advantage. You were born to be my
reader. You will not disappoint me.

While I cannot know your future, you can, if you care to,
know my past. It will be easy for you to know what I
looked like at any stage—there are plenty of photographs.
You can pick up a picture of me at age eight, at one of my
elaborate birthday celebrations, and see me with my hair
cut in a neat pageboy, wearing a broad striped tie around
my neck—the fashion of the day—and holding two fingers
over the head of a little boy standing next to me, who grins
up at me knowingly, not fooled. I have a pallid complexion,
a wide mouth, and big uneven teeth. I am not pretty, but I
have plenty of spirit, and since this is my birthday party
and there are many children here bearing gifts, I am full of
confidence. And there, in that photo bordered with yellowing Scotch tape, is me at age ten, sitting on a couch sand-

wiched between my two male cousins, whom I adore, and who tease me and adore me back. I am screeching with pleasure, my lips are bared over the crooked teeth, one arm appears waving over the shoulder of my elder cousin, one bare foot is thrust up in the air, toes blurred, blue rubber thong about to slip off. And there I am on a hilltop above Nice, on a trip to France with my parents the summer before I turn fifteen. Behind me is the sweeping crescent of the Côte d'Azur, a slice of blue water and white sand and pastel buildings. I am wearing pink short-shorts and a matching pink tube top and I am impossibly thin, my long legs tapering to a sharp point, my arms like needles. My breasts are little nubs under the stretch fabric of the top: I hardly know what to make of myself. On top of this spindly body is a leaden face, paralyzed by adolescence. All the energy and spirit of my childhood has fled.

From the age of fourteen until the age of seventeen you will find no photographs of me with my mouth open because my savage teeth are being domesticated by braces. You would get the impression that I am an unapproachable, somewhat threatening girl, whose uniformly sullen mood is sometimes enlivened by flashes of anger and raw defiance. It's the face of someone with a severe mental defect, or a serial killer. But suddenly, at eighteen, there I am again, in an entirely different mode—fake carefree, head thrown back in imitation of a fashion model, and showing lots of teeth. I am home for winter vacation after my first semester in college. I am wearing a maroon turtleneck, and a full gray skirt with a slim-fitting waist; my long hair—darker now, and wavier than it was as a child—is arranged in an elaborate upsweep; my arms are placed fearlessly akimbo. I am celebrating my liberation from high school. I have slipped into my new identity as easily as I slip into a pair of size-six jeans. If you look closely you will notice that

I am wearing way too much black eyeliner, and I will tell you a secret: I have put Vaseline on my teeth.

Next, a young woman with long streaked blond hair strides into the foreground of the photograph with a somewhat ominous air, her arms and legs arduously tanned, her expression arrogant, and also wary—this woman is a distant relative of the girl on the hilltop in Nice, a sort of third cousin twice removed. At first glance she says "touch me" but after a more considered appraisal she is still a "touch-me-not." A puzzling woman. There are many photographs to bear witness, none of them worth much, I think, because of the extreme self-awareness of the subject—her insistence on posing in full regalia, from eye make-up to high heels, for example. She is a propagandist for herself—she is determined to suppress any surfacings of the girl in Nice, who does tend to surface again in candid moments, or moments of solitude, none of which are ever permitted to be photographed. After this exhausting era is finally over, you can look at many photographs of me hiking all up and down the world with your father—my happy early thirties, my carefree years. There I am smiling over my shoulder, perched on a bench on a peak in Switzerland—muscular legs crossed, feet in big boots, the Alps soaring behind me. I am out of the photographer's studio, into nature. And, finally, there I am wearing a California poppy-yellow dress, big as a tent, with you stretching out the front until the seams are bursting.

Whenever I revisit these photographs—which I do often, mostly as an exercise in comparative identity—I am always struck by the thought that this little girl or this teenager is completely unaware of her destiny. I am fascinated by this girl's immortal bearing.

I find, however, that photographs alone are not sufficient for my purpose—my autobiographical yearnings. You could no doubt make up a whole life for me based on them, and you probably wouldn't be far off the mark either. And you might be more satisfied making up these stories than hearing somebody else's version. But I am a writer; I need words. So I have decided to tell you stories to go along with the pictures. You can draw your own conclusions after you have heard them.

A Punishment

Once upon a time, when I was eight years old, I was accused unjustly by my third grade teacher of passing notes during class and was kept after school and commanded to write twenty-five times on a piece of paper, "I will not pass notes while Miss Higgins is teaching." Miss Higgins herself sat at her desk and waited for me to complete this task, her trim ankles folded neatly, *Life* magazine flipped open on her desktop. Before she turned the pages, she would touch her left index finger to her tongue. I sat at my desk four rows from the front, slightly off-center.

Schools looked very different than they do now, Benjamin, where all the desks are arranged in friendly, encouraging circles with the children facing each other as well as the teacher, designed to foster a team spirit and to inspire students with a sense of community responsibility regarding their education. If one among you cannot multiply twelve times five, then none of you can—something like that, I suppose. When you go to kindergarten, you will witness this for yourself, and the arrangement of your classroom, and the philosophy behind this arrangement, will seem as natural to you as my classroom did then. In my childhood, schools took a more linear approach to the education of the young. We were not encouraged to look at each other, but only at the teacher who was our primary focal point throughout the long day. We, therefore, faced strictly forward. The teacher, meanwhile, most certainly did not hold forth in the center of a circle or stroll casually back and forth across the classroom, like a peripatetic classical scholar. Everybody stayed in their allotted place; as a student, it was your own business to learn what you needed to know, not anybody else's. All the desks in a column were attached—they were manufactured that way, but it is interesting to observe that although we were linked so inexorably one to the other, we could see no more of each other than the back of the head or a slice of profile.

So much of our school day was taken up by the search for distraction, and many of our distractions centered around this desk. The surface was a plastic flip-up top, under which was a compartment where you could store your textbooks and paper and wooden ruler and Elmer's glue. There was a groove on the top where you could rest a pencil and another indentation where you could rest a big square pink eraser, a requisite school supply. When we were bored in class, we had two recourses: we could rub our erasers over the plastic desk top until we had a pile of soft shavings. Or we could put a drop of Elmer's glue on our finger, wait until it dried to a hard crust, then peel it off and touch the still-gooey stuff on the inside.

The big school clock just below the American flag (we said the Pledge of Allegiance every morning) ticked peacefully. This, and the sound of Miss Higgins turning pages, and the occasional hum of a distant vacuum cleaner, were the only noises. Miss Higgins ignored me.

I had never had to stay after school before. If Miss Higgins had known anything about me, she would have known that it was impossible for me to pass notes during class, because I did not have anyone to pass notes to. I walked to school and back by myself, and at recess I sat on a bench behind the jungle gym and read *Little Women.* I would never have dreamed of breaking the rules. What had happened was this: two girls who sat on each side of me, Miriam and Jocelyn, had been passing notes to each other. Miriam leaned over to me and hissed, "Hey, pass this to Jocelyn." I shook my head, horrified. Miriam bared her teeth and raised her eyebrows and leered at me like a vampire. So I passed the note to Jocelyn, and that's when Miss Higgins spotted me.

Miss Higgins, like Miriam, had taken an unaccountable disliking to me almost as soon as I had entered her classroom at the beginning of the fall term. Or maybe not so unaccountable. I had zero to recommend me to a teacher's favor. I was pallid and solemn, with straight, sometimes greasy hair. I wore a housekey on a string around my neck, because both my parents worked; the housekey made a lump under my clothes, and if I let it hang on the outside, it clanked against my desk. Either way it was death in the classroom: the key sealed my fate. I was smart—a trait that can be irritating to teachers. I had a habit of interpreting Miss Higgins' assignments in ways that could not fail to displease her. For example, at Thanksgiving she asked us to make paper cutouts of pilgrims' hats, turkeys, and Indians to decorate the room. She specifically requested these items. Instead, I cut a large blob out of orange cardboard paper and dotted it with thick globs of Elmer's glue—I told her it was candied sweet potatoes with marshmallows. She never knew what she was going to get from me. I was subversive. My silence only made me all the more dangerous, and she was always on the lookout for me.

Miss Higgins was a sadist. I knew what this meant, without having any word to represent it yet. The first day I walked into her classroom my scalp prickled. I was a classic target for a sadist; she must have spotted me right away. I was pee-in-my-pants nervous all day long, five days a week, for the whole third grade. At the same time I had a crush on her. She was about twenty-five years old, with short dark hair and brown eyes. She wore fashionable clothes, mini-skirts and white boots and crocheted vests. I was confused by my crush and my fear and between these two emotions I was completely squashed, a miserable splotch on the clean third grade slate. Is it any wonder she didn't like me?

The clock ticked—a quarter after three. I'd been there fifteen minutes and hadn't written one of my twenty-five lines yet. Miss Higgins looked at me and said, "I'm waiting," and went back to her magazine. I studied her intensely, noticing the thin sharp bones of her ankles and the way her frosted pink lipstick was flaking. My pencil hovered over my notebook. Then, suddenly, I began to write. That was the way it always was with me—everything just poured out. I've seen pictures of myself writing. I have a hunched look, like a vulture. My elbows stick out and my left hand is twisted grotesquely, because most notebooks, with their metal binders on the left side, have been designed for right-handers. Miss Higgins smiled palely to herself. She could see that dark smudge forming on my left pinkie finger and she liked that.

At three thirty I was still writing. Miss Higgins began to look fidgety. "Aren't you done yet?" she asked.

"I'll be done in a few minutes," I replied loftily.

She got a bit twitchy at that statement. But she let it go, and at twenty to four I ripped out five notebook pages crammed with writing, shuffled up to her desk and handed them to her silently.

She took them and read, and as she read, her face blanched beneath her make-up and little waves of fury danced up and down over her features. I had not written my required twenty-five lines. Instead, I had written her a whole essay, explaining why I had been unjustly punished, and how she had deliberately misunderstood and misinterpreted the events which had occurred that day with Miriam and Jocelyn. It was an impassioned discourse. I pleaded my case eloquently and condemned her as unfair and too hasty to judge. We had studied the term "prejudice" earlier that year in the social studies section of our class, and I used the word correctly in a sentence and pointed out that she was prejudiced against me, just the way the Caucasian race was prejudiced against the Negro race. It was *Miriam and Jocelyn* she ought to punish, not me. I hinted that if she wanted me to, I could write many more pages expounding the classroom sins of these two girls, enough to get them suspended for many years. I would be glad to do this for her, if it would help her to understand that I was innocent. Miss Higgins ought to value me more and treat me with the respect I deserved. She did not seem to realize that I was one of the brightest students in the whole third grade.

Miss Higgins stood up, then sat down again, then stood up once more, catching her breath. She crumpled my essay and threw it on the floor.

"What is this?" she screeched. "What is this supposed to be?"

I was too terrified to reply. It was one thing to be bold on paper, quite another thing in the flesh.

"Just who do you think you are?" she screamed. She was getting very worked up and out of breath. "What sort of person do you think you are, that you can get away with this? How dare you *mock* me in this way?"

Ben, I had never expected my writing to fetch such a response; it was shocking. Miss Higgins' behavior was a revelation to me. I think it was in that moment that I realized the true power of the written word, and the power of the writer who wields that word. Life's unfair, but if you can write about it, you can even the score a bit. I never forgot this lesson.

"If you think you're special, you're not," she shouted. "This—this piece of trash—this means *nothing,* you hear? Maybe you have some ideas about yourself, but you better get down off your high horse, young lady, and learn how to obey your teacher."

But I knew she was wrong; I knew I was special. Who else except me could have made her rant and rave like that?

"You will sit back down at your desk and write your twenty-five lines right now. You will not leave this room until you have completed this assignment. I have plenty of time. I can wait."

I sat back down at my desk but I did not write the lines. I sat there with my head bowed over the blank page. I was pulsating with fear; I seemed to have created a monster up there. She paced and muttered to herself.

The clock ticked. It was four fifteen. Miss Higgins stood over me, slamming her fist on my notebook. "Write your lines. Write your lines." She took the pencil and tried to cram it between my limp fingers. Only, in her fury, she got the hand wrong: she tried to put it in my right hand. "You stupid little girl, *write those lines.*"

I held out until four thirty, when my mother showed up. She had come home from work and found me gone, had panicked and run next door to the neighbor's house. The neighbor's kid, who was in my class, had told her I'd been kept after school. So she'd stormed over to investigate.

My mother was a teacher herself and she was not afraid of other teachers. This was a quality I admired. She dragged Miss Higgins out into the hallway and they did battle. Miss Higgins had nearly lost her mind. "I will not be dis-obeyed!" she shouted. "I don't care if you scream to high heaven, I will not be crossed like that!"

In the end my mother must have won because she marched in and rescued me. Outside in the deserted school lot she squeezed my hand tightly and only then did I permit myself to blubber. I had been holding myself in for an hour and a half and I had really been very humiliated. But my shame was also tinged with joy. I had triumphed. To this day, I am still very proud of that essay I wrote for Miss Higgins. It was a fine piece of writing.

Faith

Here is one more old photograph that I have found, and a story to go with it. This is a story about your grandfather, who died before your third birthday, and right after my thirty-eighth. I was shocked when he died, Ben, because I thought I would be the one to die first. I do not mean to sound morbid—I only mean that as a statement of fact. I had been diagnosed two years previously with HIV. I had already been living with it, I calculated, for at least thirteen years, if not more. How much longer could I go on? People I had just gotten acquainted with had passed away in the last few months. In spite of the fact that I was healthy, thanks to the drugs, I doubted I would turn forty or live to see the twenty-first century. I had made my will; I had already decided what poetry I wanted read at my funeral— the twenty-third psalm, of course, and Shakespeare's song "Fear No More the Heat of the Sun," and Emily Dickinson and John Donne. My father would be seventy-seven in a few months, and he had throat cancer. Still, I never dreamed it would be his funeral I would be planning.

I understood that my father was mortal. But I did not believe he was mortal in the way other people were mortal: because he was my father, and I needed him, it seemed natural

that he would stay around for as long as I continued to
need him and would not even think of dying. People I knew
in their forties and even their fifties still had their fathers.
But even that was just some arbitrary cutoff point that I did
not think really applied to me. When I thought of the age I
would have to be before I allowed my father to surrender to
death, I was much older than fifty—I was an old lady myself in my imagination, even older than my father, ninety-
five, a hundred maybe. But, somehow, my father would still
be there, to comfort me through the indignities of old age
the way he had comforted me through childhood illnesses
and my present illness. It seemed quite clear to me that I
would need my father until I too died and therefore his own
death would have to be postponed indefinitely. We never
discussed this; it was something I thought we had agreed
upon long ago, when I was just a child, and did not need to
talk about. Yet in spite of this understanding between us, he
died anyhow. No apologies, no excuses—he just died.

The place is Cape Cod. I am four years old, and I am wearing a bright-red hooded sweatshirt over my bathing suit
bottoms, which are ruffled, like a skirt. I am leaning against
a railing, one foot on the ground, one foot up, in a jaunty
pose; behind me is our motel, and behind that, there is a
beige stretch of sand and a hint of the ocean. I am grinning.
My happiness is born of restored confidence in the sanity
and goodness of the world. You would never have guessed
that not long before that photograph was taken, I had been
sobbing inconsolably. Next to the picture of me is pasted a
picture of my father, holding a large beach ball in his arms
that almost obscures his narrow chest. He, too, is all grins:
our two faces seem to reflect one another, and they are very
much alike. We both have small noses, wide mouths, and

toothy smiles. He has a darker complexion than I do, and thicker eyebrows, and he is a man and much older, but, nevertheless, the happiness we share makes us twins. His joy springs from the same source as mine: faith in the absolute rightness of the universe.

That morning I had been playing on the beach. It could not have been a warm day, and probably there was a breeze—that would explain the red hooded sweatshirt. The ball I was kicking and tossing in the air had been inflated by my father—one of the tasks that always seemed to fall to him naturally. (How many hundreds of balloons, balls, and rafts did he blow up over the course of my childhood?) It was low tide, and sandbars stretched as far as the horizon. My mother had warned me to stay back from the edge of the water, but I had disobeyed her and was hopping in my bare feet on the squishy wet sand. The ball was so large it was hard for me to get both arms around it, and it kept bouncing away from me, just out of reach. Then, suddenly, a rough breeze rose up and snatched it, carrying it far out over the water. The malice of this action! I was thrown off balance, equilibrium destroyed. The ball landed in one of the shallow tide pools, and for a moment it looked like it was wavering between the shore and the temptation of the water beyond. It succumbed, and the breeze lifted it still farther and it rolled lightly over each sandbar until it was so far out of sight I could barely see it anymore.

When my father heard me crying, he took off running. He did not say to me, "Don't worry, we'll buy you another ball," or, worse, "It's just a ball, honey." He simply took off. I looked at him in amazement—I had never seen him run so fast. He plunged into the shallow water and kept on running, zigzagging and hopping over stones and sandbars in pursuit of the beach ball.

My mother and I watched him. Sometimes it seemed like

he was gaining on the ball, sometimes it seemed like the malevolent forces of the universe were going to win. Often my father had to cross patches of water that were up to his chest—and he did not know how to swim. He became a stick figure on the horizon—a slight man with spindly legs chasing a ball.

And then, miraculously, he caught up with it. He held it over his head and waved it in the air; for a moment, I feared that in his exuberance he might drop it again.

He returned to shore, still running, growing larger and larger until the stick figure turned into my flesh-and-blood father again. He was out of breath; the soles of his feet were bleeding from the rough stones. But he was grinning and he looked inexpressibly happy. I met him with an answering joy. The photographs were taken immediately after that.

Ben, in that moment I understood that I had a happy childhood. My father knew all too well (and I was just beginning to learn) how precarious life is, and he must have wanted me to feel, at least for a few brief years, that I had a protector.

Much later, when I was an adult, my father rescued another precious object for me. It was only a few months after I had been diagnosed, and I felt fragile and clumsy all at once, as if my body were locked in an endless cycle of smashing things and being smashed. I had forgotten how to move, how to negotiate my way through time and space.

I owned a little black and white porcelain dog that I had been given by my great aunt, my father's Aunt Nell, someone I'd loved very much as a child. I treasured this legacy from her. The dog had moved with me from apartment to apartment, and I had kept it intact for many years. But now, I could keep nothing intact—I made one of my stupid clumsy gestures and the dog fell to the floor and shattered. I swept the pieces into a plastic bag but I did not really believe they could be put together again. I could hardly bear to look at the bag but I couldn't bring myself to throw it out either, so I hid it in a closet. A few days later, my father, noticing that I was glum, asked me what was the matter. So I showed him the fragments in the bag and he told me that he could put them back together. And he did. Miraculously, he returned with the little dog made almost whole again—minus an ear, and sticky with glue, but, nonetheless, recognizable. He was quietly pleased with himself, but even more pleased when he saw the joy I felt at having the dog returned to me in nearly its original state. Once again my father had put things right for me, or as right as it was in his power to do so. He knew that he could not cure my illness or end my pain, but he never doubted the worth of small acts of kindness, or his ability to perform them.

Clairvoyance

This time we are on another vacation, on another cape: Cape Hatteras, off the coast of North Carolina. I am six years old. A great storm is brewing on the Atlantic seaboard.

Ben, I am more fortunate than you, because I was already a young adult before any of the members of my family died. You, having the ill luck to be born to parents who were no longer young themselves, and whose own parents were elderly, have had to suffer through the deaths of your maternal grandfather and your paternal grandmother, all before the age of four. You were forced to develop an early awareness of death: when your grandfather passed away, you asked me, "Where did Papa go?" and you have had to make do the best you can with my inept and insufficient reply: "Nobody knows. I believe he's still all around us, and inside us." Once you digested this puzzling information, you expounded upon it, so that a year later, when your Grandmother Myrtle died, you were ready: "If Grandmother Myrtle is inside me, can she see what goes into my stomach when I eat?" or "Does it bother Grandmother Myrtle when I go down the slide in the playground? Maybe she doesn't like to be bounced." You were also concerned about the space the dead occupy: "Is there room for Papa *and* Grandma Myrtle inside me?"

It was time to explain to you the theory of the body's separation from the spirit. You seemed to absorb it smoothly, although you still had your doubts: "If Grandma Myrtle is buried, how can she tell when it's morning?" (Your Grandma Myrtle was not buried. May God forgive me for telling you this small lie.)

It was not long before you made the great leap from comprehending that two beloved people in your life had died to comprehending that *all* of us must die. And of course, that *you* must die. First and foremost you were concerned about yourself. "When will I die?" you asked anxiously and when we gave you the standard response, "Not for a long, long time," it was not nearly concrete enough for you, and you demanded to know, "Will I live to be one hundred and fifty-five? Will I live to be two thousand and eighty-two?" You wanted to know how long everything would live—trees, airplanes, stones, your fire truck. Eventually—you approached the topic ever so cautiously, from an oblique angle—you asked when your father would die, and when I would die.

I would rather have walked over hot coals in my bare feet than had to answer such questions. But you deserved an answer. So I devised one that I hoped was not too dissembling or falsely optimistic, that combined just the right measures of truth and balm. (Parenthood involves one grand deception, Ben: we deceive our children into believing that we know exactly where we're heading.) With regard to your father, I replied, "Daddy is very healthy and will probably live a long, long time." With regard to myself, I modified the response slightly: "Mommy is in good health right now and hopefully she will live a long time too." I prayed fervently that these replies might lay your anxieties to rest.

Ben, you were smarter than I gave you credit for, and you immediately registered the subtle discrepancies in these answers. You had seen me take pills morning, noon, and night, and now you demanded to know what they were for. Once again stumbling about in the dark, I told you, "Mommy has a bug inside of her that won't go away. But the pills keep her healthy so she can play with you and have lots of fun!" The high-pitched, false joviality of the addended last phrase disgusted me, but, miraculously, it worked: you were diverted, at least for the time being, from the contemplation of your mother's mortality.

Still, although you rarely question me anymore, I know that your anxiety has burrowed its way under your skin, that it often reveals itself in your nervous tics, your tendency to scratch and sometimes bite yourself, and your sudden squalls of violence. You were just an infant when my illness manifested itself, and since then, to all outward appearances, I have been just a normal mommy like any other mommy on the block, but I have no doubt that what you witnessed as a baby remains with you, like film waiting in the darkroom to be developed. I was younger than you are now when I watched my own mother writhing in agony on the living room couch, and my father comforting her as they waited for the ambulance to come. Her Fallopian tube pregnancy precluded our small family from growing any larger—just as my illness has put a stop to any more childbearing of my own—but I would have sacrificed dozens of brothers and sisters in order to erase the memory of my mother's suffering from my mind. That scene stays with me forever, it's part of psyche and soul, and I've learned to co-exist with it, just as you, Benjamin, will have to learn to co-exist with your memories of your own mother's sickbed. God knows I'd wrench them out of your mind if I could.

Back now to Cape Hatteras and the hurricane, for a hurricane it was, although we did not guess that at first, because our car radio was on the blink. I'm telling you this tale because your ruminations about death reminded me of a strange premonition that visited me more than thirty years ago.

We drive and drive and drive to reach the cabin we have rented. Cape Hatteras is a wild deserted place, and from my position strapped in the back seat of the car, it looks like nothing but dunes and eerie swaying grasses and telephone poles. It goes on like this for miles. Although the car windows are closed, the loneliness of the place seeps through the cracks, and it seeps into me. My inside loneliness becomes all mixed up with this outside loneliness and it frightens me. I don't know what is me anymore, or what is Cape Hatteras. I feel as if I am losing myself inch by inch; helpless, I watch myself, a little girl with a blue butterfly-shaped barrette in her hair, climbing up a dune, teetering slightly at the rise, then disappearing, swallowed by the great gaping horizon. I am gone; disintegrated. I and the cape and the loneliness are all part of the same thing now. Inside of me—where I once knew for certain that I could always find myself, in the space I had always occupied—there is a gigantic hollowness. Winds rush in and out of me as if I am a drafty cavern. I am at their mercy.

Something terrible is happening on Cape Hatteras, but I seem to be the only one who notices this. I look over the top of the front seat and see my parents talking to each other as if nothing out of the ordinary is happening. I use all my will power to contain myself, because I know this is our vacation, and it means a lot to my parents, who work very hard and have been looking forward to coming to the ocean.

Finally we arrive at our cabin, one of a few that are studded along a strip of the dunes. Ours is the only car in the parking lot. It is early afternoon, but the sky is laden with clouds; their bellies sag in the water. Everything is a strange pewter color—the water, the sky, the sand. My mother and I venture over the boardwalk to the beach, while my father unloads the bags from our car. We stand there tentatively, looking at the dubious landscape. The sand is dark and sodden. Gleaming strips of black seaweed stripe the beach in horizontal lines. An old Twinkies wrapper and a cigarette butt are ground into the sand near my feet. A few yards away, the mutilated remains of a seagull. It's the first dead creature I've ever seen. The wind picks up and the Twinkies wrapper is yanked away; there is a strange humming noise I can't identify.

I know things. We are so small, the three of us, my dear mother and father and me, and there is no way we can survive. Things die and disappear forever, never to be seen again. The planet Earth that we live on is so enormous it is incomprehensible, but even it is very small and is whirling away, beyond our control, in the still larger sky. I know these things in spite of the fact that, up until a second before when I spotted the seagull, I had never had an inkling of death, never lost a close relative or a friend, as I told you.

Suddenly I have a sort of premonition, that's the only way I know how to describe it, Ben. I am lying flat on my back, enclosed on all sides by wooden boards that are only an inch or two away from my arms and legs and the tip of my nose. It is dark and silent, except for a faint tapping. I am in a coffin (although I have never seen or heard of such a thing before, that is what it is). I am about to be buried many feet underground, but I am not dead—not yet. I can move; I lift my hand and place it flat against the damp underside of the lid, coming away with a splinter. Somehow, although the fact of being in a coffin is frightening from a rational point of view, in another, deeper sense, it is strangely comforting. I feel embraced, protected in this small space where there is no room for either expansion or error. I think I will lie there quietly and dream about something—what doesn't seem to matter. But the tapping sound annoys me; it won't let me rest. Tap, tap, tap, on it goes, just above my head, as grating as a leaky faucet. Gradually I begin to realize that the tapping sound is meant for me—someone is trying to determine whether I am alive, whether they should pry open the coffin and release me. They are waiting for me to tap back. I could easily do so—in fact, I place my fingers against the roof, in preparation, but I do not move them to make a sound.

Now, and only now, I begin to get scared. What felt womblike before now makes me feel wildly claustrophobic. I know that if I don't let someone know I am here, I will be buried for good, and I am desperate to get out. But I'm not at all sure that my fingers will obey me. I listen to the tapping grow fainter until it almost disappears and I urge my fingers to move, but they are paralyzed. They have a will of their own. Tap, please tap, I pray. There's not much time left. Yet something prevents them. I don't trust my hands to save me and that is just as terrifying as the idea of being buried alive.

Never fear, Ben, the story has a happy ending—your mother, in the final analysis, no matter how seductive it is to remain silent, will always give a tap so she can be heard. And that is just what I do in this strange waking dream—I put my heart into it, I screw up all the courage I have, I force my hands to work again, and I pound my fists against the coffin's lid. In that moment I am released from the grip of the presentiment.

Then I begin to sob—retching, heaving sobs. I fall to my knees in the damp sand. I howl and tremble. My mother throws her entire body on top of me to smother out whatever it is that's possessed me. She hunches over me and I make myself very small and tight underneath her. My father runs toward her from the cabin. He has heard on the motel's radio that a hurricane is expected to hit the cape that night. We toss all our still-packed bags into the trunk, climb into the car, and drive away from Cape Hatteras.

Thirty years later, during the summer when I am sick and cannot figure out what is wrong with me, I have the exact same waking dream—the coffin, the tapping, the immobilized hands. Even while I am having the dream I realize that the only other time in my life that I have ever had such a bizarre experience was when I was six years old, on Cape Hatteras, during a hurricane.

Passion

First thing, Ben, find out what it is you love.

When I was ten and a half years old, I fell madly in love with my friend Goldie's typewriter. I had never seen one before, but the moment I set eyes on it, I knew that I was meant to possess it, or at least one very like it. I am afraid that I valued her typewriter more than I valued her and that I was guilty of some duplicity in my relationship with her. I pretended to enjoy her company just so that I could be near her machine. I frequently insinuated myself into her house on the pretext of needing to use the bathroom, and sometimes, feeling desperate, I shamelessly invited myself over to

play. She herself did not place half such a value on the typewriter; she rarely touched it. How in the world could she
have kept her hands off of it, I wondered? Her room was
the neatest I'd ever seen. Sometimes when I was visiting, her
mother would enter her room without knocking and would
proceed to brush all the objects on Goldie's desk and her
bookcase with a green feather duster, moving soundlessly
across the room on her miniature feet. Then she would disappear again, without a word.

The typewriter, a Smith Corona portable, sparkled on
Goldie's desk. It had a handsome reddish brown cover,
which, when removed, revealed a machine without parallel
in the universe, as far as I was concerned. The typebars with
their raised letters were shiny and untarnished by age or
ink. Straight and snappy, they sprang against the platen
with a quick tap when you pressed the corresponding key
below, always true to the mark. The ribbon was still a virgin black, rich and deep, threaded to perfection through the
spools. When you pushed the carriage return, a merry bell
rang out triumphantly. Goldie had been given the typewriter as a Hanukkah present, because her father was a
German-Jew who believed that children should be offered
practical gifts. I gave him credit for not having bought her a
"child's" typewriter, made of cheap pink or blue plastic,
with extra-large keys or, worse, Disney figures painted on
the cover. This was the real thing. But Goldie remained un-
moved by the typewriter's tantalizing possibilities. It
amazed me that something I coveted could be viewed by
another human being as merely another inanimate object.

I used to approach her desk with my heart pounding. My
fingers brushed the keys, which I would feel give ever so
lightly beneath me, responding to my tentative touch. Then
I would grow bolder, and insert a crisp white sheet of paper
into the roller—in those days, Ben, there was no more

beautiful sight in the world to me than a fresh piece of 8½-by-11 typewriter paper. I puzzled over the mystery of the keyboard, why the letters were scattered instead of laid out in correct alphabetical order. But I accepted the universe of the typewriter without question. I typed words with one finger—first my name and then Goldie's name, and then, warming up to it, any words that occurred to me—"fecund," "preposterous," "alleviate," "justifiably," and "invigorate." It was the fact that the machine produced *words* which enthralled me. The words that bloomed in my head were instantaneously reproduced on the page. It was the most seductive thing: irresistible.

But it took me a long time to type words with one finger and Goldie would grow restless waiting for me to finish. She would whine for me to play Clue or Life or gin rummy with her. Eventually we quarreled and I was cut off from her typewriter and I realized that it was imperative that I acquire a typewriter of my own. And so I began begging my parents. I was systematic: I begged at breakfast, before my parents left for work, and I begged when my mother came home from teaching in the late afternoon, and I put in some additional begging at dinner, when both my mother and my father were at the table. Ben, your mother is the type of person whose original motives are often eroded by self-doubt, but on rare occasions in my life—and this was one of them—I have understood that my desires have taken on a life of their own, that my shyness is immaterial to them, and I have been uncharacteristically tenacious about satisfying them. It is I who am serving them, not the other way around. Being under the influence of such carnivorous desires was almost a transcendental experience. But it didn't happen often.

And so, for my eleventh birthday, I was presented with a typewriter. Not a Smith Corona, but a good serviceable

Sears Roebuck manual portable. Perhaps not as flashy as Goldie's, but far dearer to me because it was my own. My mother offered to pay for typing lessons, but I smiled and showed her the book I had purchased in anticipation of my birthday present—a slim workbook entitled *How to Type in Ten Easy Lessons.*

Almost every morning I would wake up at six A.M. and practice for two hours before I had to go to school. I sprang out of bed at six A.M. on the weekends also, and immediately began banging away. Manual typewriters were noisy, and I was enthusiastic with the carriage return and the bell. I'm sure my parents' sleep must have been disturbed, but if it was, they never said anything. They loved me and wanted me to be happy. And I *was* happy divining the mysteries of the typewriter. I learned how to rest my fingers lightly, poised for action, on the center row of "home" keys, and I memorized the letters under each finger's domain. Once memorized, I never forgot those things: they became a part of my existence as intimate and integral as my skin or my veins. I dutifully practiced every one of the workbook exercises—from short sentences about taking proper phone messages to three-paragraph instructions regarding the importance of dressing correctly for a job interview in the typing pool. I learned how to set tabs and margins, how to backspace, how to change the ribbon, how to minimize the chance of errors. In those days there were no "correction" keys, no automatic erasure. You had to use a white liquid to blot out the offensive letter or word, wait patiently for it to dry, then backspace and carefully type over it, hoping that it would not be smudged or sticky. And if you wanted to insert new words or paragraphs onto the page, you simply had to type it all over again. Most people typed from a handwritten manuscript, and so what you typed had to be in its final stages—it was a more serious business than typing on a computer screen, where you could be more cavalier about mistakes. There was something uniquely exciting about the typewriter because it represented the thrill of the finished product, the next best thing to print itself. A computer screen is more fluid, more process than achievement. You really did feel, after you had typed a paper (they were not called "documents" in those days), that you had reached some kind of fruition. I am sorry, Ben, that you yourself will never experience the sensation of using a typewriter; you were born square in the middle of the computer age, and typewriters are virtually obsolete. Only curmudgeons and collectors hang onto them now.

In six weeks I had learned how to type. In all the time I had been under the spell of the typewriter, I had never once questioned why I had been driven to type in the first place. It seems to me, in looking back, that I wanted to type because I wanted to write. Even though I had a box full of stories, poems, and plays written in longhand, I must have believed that validation as a writer could only be arrived at through typing. And it's true that after I learned how to type, I began to write voraciously—much more voraciously than I ever wrote on a computer. In sheer volume alone my output was astonishing, and I was never again in my life able to match the rollicking pace I achieved at the ages of eleven, twelve, and thirteen. Everything I wrote seemed wondrous to me, and I would peer adoringly at the growing pile of pages in my desk drawer.

I also put my typing to more practical use. I earned some pocket money typing papers for my mother, who was returning to school at night to get her master's degree. We would both sit at the dining room table and she would spread out her anguished drafts—pages renumbered, insertions, big X's blacking out whole sections, coffee stains and ink smudges everywhere. She could not write a paper without doubting herself, turning back, and writing it all over again before she had finished even a first version. She would read the pages out loud to me, getting the order mixed up, dictating a paragraph only to cry, "No! Wait a minute! That should have been on page three!" She was killing herself. During all this, I remained cool, fingers poised in waiting over the home keys, superior as only an eleven year old can be with regard to her parent's failings. I charged her a dollar a page, quite a lot of money in those days. She could have hired a professional typist, but she preferred to keep the whole shameful proceeding in the family, so she paid me what I wanted. And anyway, I was almost as good as a professional typist. My typing skills were legendary in the sixth grade.

My first Sears Roebuck typewriter lasted through my second year of high school. Toward the end of its life, it looked nothing like Goldie's typewriter, the typewriter that had first inspired me. The typebars were gnarled and disfigured; half of them were stuck and could no longer reach the page. The keys—what was left of them—were slick with grease. Cookie crumbs, bits of peanut butter sandwiches, splashes of juice had fallen into the spaces between them. The carriage bell had long since stopped ringing; the ribbon was dotted with holes. The typewriter had seen hundreds upon hundreds of pages pass through its roller, and it was spent. Technology was beginning to pass it up too. Still, it was a mistake to get rid of it. I would like to have it today, to show it to you, Ben, and to bear witness to my youthful passion.

Sustenance

Phyllis was a cleaning lady who worked for us when I was nine years old. She was the first adult, aside from family members, who liked me just for myself. We took to each other right away. When she arrived at our house the first time, I was in the middle of a screaming match with my mother—"Why did you throw away that piece of cardboard—that was going to be the drawbridge for Barbie's castle!" Phyllis stood back coolly, arms crossed, appraising me. Then she said to my mother, admiringly, "That girl is *hard-headed*." I took a good look at her too: a statuesque black woman in her late twenties, wearing leopard-skin stretch pants, a shimmery gold tunic, and mules. She had a big bosom. Her heels were worn smooth and yellow; her toes and fingernails were painted a fiery orange. Her hair, which had been elaborately straightened and teased, added two inches to her height. She reminded me of my beloved aunt, a woman about the same age who would show up for her semiannual visits wearing white go-go boots and a green feather boa. I liked a flashy woman. I had aspirations in that direction myself.

Once a week Phyllis would arrive just before I left for school, and she would be there to make me lunch at noontime. (The other days, I ate at a friend's house.) It's anybody's guess what her duties consisted of before I came home—probably laundry, dishes, some dusting and vacuuming. Her housekeeping skills were indifferent at best, because, in spite of her hours of labor, I never remember our house being any cleaner. The vacuum cleaner bag remained suspiciously empty after months of use, and after a year in our service, the oven was still thickly coated with grease. But her uselessness as a housekeeper couldn't have mattered less to me. Or to my mother either. Cleaning wasn't exactly the point—it had started out to be, but Phyllis's function had evolved into something different.

This was the 1960s, and my mother had problems keeping cleaning ladies, not because she was tyrannical or

demanding, but just the opposite: she felt guilty and didn't
have any idea how to coexist with someone you had hired
to scrub your toilet. She'd grown up in a poor family and
now, in this inflammatory era of civil rights battles, Mal-
colm X, integration and student riots, she was even more
confused. But she taught fulltime and she was no kind of
cleaner herself; although she wasn't overly fussy, she understood that *someone* had to clean. But she was tortured by
the "who." So we had cleaning ladies. We had *dozens* of
cleaning ladies, as a consequence of my mother's insecur-
ities. I used to envy friends who talked about their "Almas"
or their "Mays," women who had been cleaning for their
families when my friends were still in diapers, women who
came on a regular day at a regular time, week in and week
out, year after year. Women who received birthday presents
from my friend's families and who, when they went to visit
their relatives in El Salvador or Guatemala once a year for
three weeks, would faithfully send their nieces to clean in
their place.

I hated getting used to the new ladies. My mother experimented with all shapes, sizes, colors, and creeds. She had
the hardest time assimilating "Negroes"—the acceptable
term in those days—into her household. Not out of any
kind of prejudice or fear; no, it was because a Negro hired
to work for you only served to broadcast the vast discrepancy between the social classes, not to mention the ugly
specter of racism. Any kind of Hispanic immigrant was also
out of the question for many of the same reasons, but also
because as a rule they were so warm-hearted, so tender in
nature, as to be almost intolerable. Eastern Europeans—
Czechs, Hungarians, Romanians, Poles—were preferable.
Poles were the best of all because they were notoriously
anti-Semitic, and this made my mother feel more comfortable giving them orders. She didn't have to feel guilty about

hiring them as underlings: the lines of demarcation had been drawn long ago, and there was no nonsense about equality and civil rights when you were dealing with Poles. But the Polish cleaning women were, for the most part, aggressive, obstreperous, and uncommunicative and my mother, for all her eagerness to hire them, almost always found them to be unmanageable once she'd gotten them in the house. White college girls and white housewives trying to make some extra money while their kids were in school should have been ideal, but they made my mother uneasy because they were almost too familiar: it was as if she had hired a niece or a cousin.

I was to blame for the loss of a few cleaning ladies also. Your mother, Ben, was never a docile child, quiet reputation notwithstanding. I did not express myself in bounces, as you do, but I had a great deal of cunning and verbal pyrotechnics at my disposal. Poor Mrs. Barromeo, a frail, patrician Bolivian woman, quaked under the volley of curses I pelted at her after she had rearranged my dollhouse furniture while dusting. And there was Mrs. O'Riley: while she was on her hands and knees scouring the kitchen linoleum, I crept up and scribbled on her large behind with magic markers. By the time Phyllis strode so elegantly into our lives my mother was almost defeated and I was cynical. But Phyllis had both our numbers. She had some sterling qualities to recommend her as a cleaning lady: chief among them were disdain, a well-developed sense of irony, and a healthy portion of self-esteem. She made my mother feel as if she was doing her a favor cleaning her house. My mother was relieved: at last, help you could rely on.

Phyllis had nothing but contempt for my mother's housekeeping. She filled my ears with vehement complaints during lunch, that hour when we cemented our friendship: "Girl, how can I dust if your mother leaves all that junk

piled everywhere? Books, newspapers a month old, cata-
logues, apple cores. I'm not allowed to throw anything out.
That isn't my job, is it? Most homes, the lady does some
straightening up before her help comes. That's only fair. But
in all my days I've never *seen* a house like this. There's no
order anywhere. You ask her where something belongs, she
gets that funny look on her face—you know what I'm talking about—then she gets that scared tone in her voice and
she says, 'I don't know,'" Phyllis snorted. "I don't know!
You ever heard of anything like that? How can you not
know where something belongs in your own house? I guess
she must be a smart lady since she's a school teacher and
all, but just between you and me, she doesn't have one
ounce of common sense."

My mother's furniture also failed to live up to Phyllis's
standards. "Nothing matches," she complained. "Why
can't your mother go down to Wards and buy herself a nice
armchair and sofa that belong together?"

She let it be known that she had cleaned much better
quality houses than ours, real homes with rugs that were
bought new instead of from a garage sale, homes with dish-
washers (she hinted at this many times) and food process-
ing machines. I understood that she only cleaned our house
out of charity. If her attentions were indifferent at best, that
was our fault. What could a charity case expect?

But there was one thing she did do superlatively, and she
did it just for me. When I came home for lunch, she always
made me French fries. And what French fries! They were
her masterpiece, and they were my weekly joy. Since then
I've never found their equal, not even in the fanciest bar
and grills, and certainly not in any homemade version. She
must have served me some other lunch as well—maybe a
hamburger, a hot dog—but that was only a token gesture

and we both knew it. The French fries, Phyllis's beautiful, aromatic French fries, were the heart of the matter.

On Wednesdays I would fly home, and the moment I opened the door, my mouth began to water. I was greeted with the smell of hot oil and the rank odor of raw potatoes. Phyllis rose from her seat in the kitchen, where she had been listening to jazz music on the radio and flipping through my mother's old copies of *Vogue,* and called out joyfully, "I got 'em ready for you, baby, I'm just about to drop 'em in."

The sink was piled with potato peelings; Phyllis's perfectly cut fries, never too thick or too thin, their ends squared neatly, lay stacked on a plate to the left of the pot. She always waited until I was seated at the table before she dropped the potatoes in the hot oil—partly because she knew I loved the sizzle, partly because she insisted that fries had to be eaten straight away. Timing was crucial. If they were fried too soon before they were eaten, they lost their potency. They drooped, were less than they should be. Phyllis aimed to dazzle.

They were steaming when Phyllis heaped them on my plate, a pale gold the color of wintry sunshine, slender and succulent. Never were they a mite more greasy than they should be; Phyllis was a past master at frying, and she had a special method of shaking them as she lifted them from the pot in their mesh container. She turned up her nose, though, at spreading them on brown paper first—a French-fried potato should go straight from pot to plate, with no stages in between. Blotting was the crutch of a poor cook.

I would dip my head into the steam, letting it cloud my eyes and moisten my forehead and the tip of my nose. The moment before the first bite was so delicious I wanted it to last forever. But I only had an hour, and the French fries were not immortal, and, alas, neither was I. Phyllis hovered over me, anxious for consummation. I bit. The delicate crust crinkled between my teeth; the moist, pulpy inside filled my mouth, burning my tongue, driving out all other sensations and taking complete possession of me. How did she do it? Every fry was a work of art.

I acquired a more sophisticated palate under Phyllis's charge. On those lunch hours I learned to eschew one of my favorite foods, catsup. She did not teach me this in so many words, but I quickly discovered that the tangy-sweet flavor of that ubiquitous condiment could easily overpower the subtle aroma and flavor of the fries. They were better savored with salt, which I used liberally, urged on by Phyllis. When I was done with one plate, she would bring me another batch, not a moment too late or too soon.

While I ate, we talked. Phyllis was interested in my life— the details mattered to her. When I went out at recess, did I play on the jungle gym or on the swings? Why? Did I play with three or four other girls or just one? When she learned that I sometimes traded comic books, she wanted to know which ones. She enjoyed hearing stories about my teachers, and often asked what they were wearing that day, and laughed hard and long when I mimicked them, which I was good at.

When I was in a sullen mood she knew it and could draw out the cause, skillfully, like a surgeon with a lancet.

"What's wrong with you today? You all mush-faced."

"I'm not."

"Yes you are. Miss mush-faced. Something must have happened today in that Mr. Jellybean's class."

I laughed with my mouth full. Mr. Jellybean was the name we'd given to my math teacher because he always wore candy-colored shirts—pink, neon green, orange.

"Oh, see, I'm right then. That Mr. Jellybean marked you down on your long division again."

"There's nothing wrong with my long division."

"You can't divide anything, girl, long or short. Don't try to fool me. I know math's not your strong point."

"It wasn't that."

"Oh now I'm losing my patience. Get on back to school, then! Nobody wants to eat lunch staring at your mush face. You take away my appetite."

"It's that girl, Eleanor Sosewitz. This morning in the hallway she punched me. For no reason. She just walked up to me with some of her friends while I was getting a drink of water at the fountain and when I stood up she punched me, hard, in the shoulder."

"Nobody punches nobody for no reason. Were you sassing her or something?"

"No, I swear, I wasn't. I didn't say a word to her. I think she just hates me because I know all the answers when the teacher calls on me in social studies. Like yesterday I knew what the capital of Peru was, you know, stuff like that. She just hates me because I'm smarter than she is but she's bigger than I am so she can punch me out."

Phyllis reclined in her chair, contemplated me, rolled her eyes and snorted. She was already acquainted with Eleanor Sosewitz, through my descriptions of her: she knew, as well as I did, that Eleanor was a heavyset, bull-jawed girl who sat in the back of the class, sometimes smelled bad, and had an older brother who'd done time in jail for stealing cars. Phyllis had Eleanor Sosewitz sized up.

"Girl, you got to *not* have all the answers. You got too many of them. Next time that social studies teacher asks what the capital of Iowa is or where is Timbuktu, you keep your mouth shut, you hear? Keep it clamped shut. There's always going to be kids hate you for what you got. So what you have to do, you have to hide what you got. That's the smart way—you think you're smart, but you ain't so smart as you think, no girl, you don't know the half of what you should. What you got to always be the teacher's pet for? Okay, that's what you want, then you're going to spend your life getting punched at the water fountain. Be cool. You can be smart for the teachers and at the same time smart for yourself too. Don't let kids like Eleanor Sosewitz think you think you're better than them. Act like you're just one of them, see? But you know better and the teachers know better too. Only that's your secret. You get it? You *put the brakes* on that showing off."

By the time my lunch hour was over, I must have consumed at least three or four potatoes; my stomach was warm, full, distended, tight and round as a miniature soccer ball. Those adults who had always known me as a "poor eater" would have been surprised to see me. Phyllis's fries sustained me throughout the afternoon at school, giving me strength and courage, their weight in my belly proof that I was loved and cared for.

I don't know why Phyllis stopped working for us after a year. Perhaps she found a better position; perhaps she found a man to support her so she wouldn't have to work. It's possible my mother decided to liberate herself from cleaning ladies altogether—after all, she was rarely able to achieve the peace of mind you are supposed to achieve from a spotless, well-ordered house. The cleaner the house, the worse her guilt, and so, the worse her mental state. Whatever the reason, by the time I was ten, Phyllis was gone. I moved on to other people, other foods: she was out of my life.

She came back to visit just once, when I was twelve. I don't know if she and my mother had been keeping in touch or if, one day, on a whim, she simply rang our doorbell unannounced. Probably the latter. In any case, one summer afternoon, she appeared, and she was soon seated in the living room with my mother, drinking iced tea and talking and laughing in her full-throated way. I knew she was in the house, but I didn't want to come out of my room. I was sitting at my beloved typewriter, writing my first novel. (You will recall, Ben, that I was in the first throes of a long romance with that machine.) I had been working on it every day for weeks, ever since school let out. It was about a wealthy man named Cornelius who lived in an enormous country mansion in England. Interestingly, it was the hierarchy of servants that most enthralled me; my inspiration had been Amy Vanderbilt's fascinating and unintentionally anthropological study, *The Complete Book of Etiquette,* in which she described in painstaking detail the duties of almost every kind of "domestic." I was completely under its spell, and as I read about the subtle distinctions between a valet and a footman, or the specific spheres of influence exercised by a housekeeper and where they intersected with the spheres of the butler, my characters took shape, acquired names and personalities.

Since I was unwilling to come to her, Phyllis came to me. She knocked on my door. I opened it with the greatest reluctance. There she stood, looking the same as ever—robust, with her pronounced, curvaceous figure, her shiny black hair subjugated into a glamorous pageboy, her nails manicured within an inch of her life. She had a little boy with her, expensively dressed in ecru linen shorts and a matching short-sleeved shirt. He looked as if he defied anybody to find a wrinkle on him. She introduced him to me as her nephew, Tyrone. Then she said they were going out for ice cream and would I like to join them.

Far away as I was with Cornelius and his house full of servants, I must have been annoyed by the blatancy, the immediacy of Phyllis and Tyrone. The shock of being called back—for we are always called back, sooner or later—was more than I could tolerate at the moment. Still, that's no excuse for my behavior. I smiled at her in a chilly way (in just the manner that Cornelius's butler, Fenworth, would handle a door-to-door salesman, for example) and replied, "I can't right now, it would disturb my train of thought." She gave a staccato laugh—think of that child who used to stuff her face full of French fries having a train of thought!—and beat a quick retreat, closing the door behind her.

In the years since, Ben, I have often wondered what observations Phyllis would have made about different milestones in my life—my choice of studies at college, my marriage, my decampment to San Francisco. And of course, about the present state of affairs. I would not like to see her face if I told her I had HIV. Probably her expression would be an unholy mixture of sorrow, skepticism, belligerence, incrimination, and reluctant sympathy. It would be unbearable. Probably she would have blurted out, as most people are too timid or too well-bred to do, "How the hell did you get *that*?" And a few minutes later, "Unn-huh, girl, I *told* you so." After all, once she had warned me against vanity and pride, cautioned me not to put myself forward, not to grab the limelight, or I would suffer the consequences. She might have seen HIV as one of these consequences: "If you'd only listened . . ."

After the first shock, though, Phyllis would not waste much time with scolding and accusations. She would offer fresh advice for this fresh dilemma. "Baby, you just got to keep on stepping," is what I think she would have said. I would like to hear her say it; I'm heartily sorry now that I cast her away so thoughtlessly.

Knock on my door again, Phyllis, and invite me out for ice cream, and I'll give you the right answer this time.

The Faraway Park

Hannah Krempel, where are you? I hope not still entombed in Orthodox Judaism, stiffly wigged, a heavy broadcloth skirt swirling darkly around your ankles, your stride impeded by the hands of five or six children, born in as many years, entwining your waist and thighs. I hope not, but I fear it. In the end, everybody reverts to type. I knew you as a child when you had been deeply imprinted upon. There's a chance you had a rebellious adolescence: only a slim one, though. Now, in your late thirties, are you restless, like me? Does your life feel like an ill-fitting dress, a little tight under the armpits, the fabric bunched up around the waist? Or, on the contrary, do you fit into your life like it was custom made? I challenge you to step forth and announce yourself: "Present!"

Like you, Ben, I was the sort of child who only had one friend at a time. Mostly I was happy playing alone, but occasionally I had a craving for sociability that I had no idea how to satisfy. Because I lived so much inside of my own head, my social skills were primitive. My timid, unschooled advances to other children must have seemed repulsive to them. I could barely manage even the simplest things—inviting a classmate over to my house to play or joining the neighbor kids in a game of hide-and-seek—and I took my failures hard, knowing that what I labored over came without any effort at all to others. So when one of my attempts panned out, I cleaved to that friend with medieval loyalty. All of my friendships were significant; none were casual. I am still that way now. I am so overjoyed when the wind blows a friend my way, that I stand ready to put my whole heart into that friendship. For this reason I am probably a better friend than many more gregarious people, who take their friends, and their ability to make friends, for granted. I am dependable; I never break engagements on a whim, I grant favors without asking for them in return, I keep in touch, I always return phone calls, I am as reciprocal as I am encouraged to be, and I never forget the details of people's lives that mean so much to them.

Hannah Krempel was one of my single, and singular, friends. Her parents were landlords; in addition to the house they inhabited, a somber barnlike structure on the corner across from the junior high school, they owned a sprawling house next door to ours that had been divided into several apartments. We used to see her father knocking on the doors on the first of each month to collect the rent. (In those days, many of the tenants paid in cash.) He was a small, compact elderly gentleman with a long white beard and a black hat. He looked, walked, and talked like an Orthodox Jew, but he had been born into an Irish Catholic family and had converted when he married Hannah's mother. His conversion had been so complete that he adapted his wife's maiden name, so that the family would not have to suffer under the moniker of O'Malley. This had all happened a long, long time ago. Now, instead of a rosary, he fingered the fringes of his *tallis*. He *davened* with *tefillin* every morning.

Hannah was an only child, like me. Her mother had been past forty when she was born, and her father was a good fifteen years older than that. Their habits and manner of dress aged them another fifteen years beyond their chronological age. They were so old that they had succeeded in virtually squashing her own youth; she was the most elderly ten year old I'd ever met. I don't know how we were introduced to each other; probably by force. Her mother discovered that there was another Jewish child in the neighborhood, dragged poor Hannah over to my house, and abandoned her there, commanding, "Play!" But, fortunately, the meeting was harmonious.

I remember Hannah as having sallow skin, plump, wormlike white fingers, long brown hair and an obsequious demeanor that it took me a long time to whittle down. She always had a faintly prunish look, like someone who has been sitting in the bath too long. She was not allowed to wear pants, only skirts, long ones, and not the fashionable "maxis" or "granny gowns" with ruffles and bold geometric patterns—hers were cheerless, dun-colored, and inevitably down at the hem because she stepped on them.

But, as you might have suspected, she possessed a rich imagination. I ferreted this out of her early in our acquaintance. We did marvelous, lascivious things with paper dolls and Barbies, things I'd never done before with anybody else. (We returned the Barbies to their boxes with twisted limbs, heads facing backwards.) We acted out stories we'd invented in our heads. When it rained or snowed, we acted out our stories in my basement or hers. But when the weather was fine, we went to the faraway park.

The faraway park belonged to Hannah and to me, no matter how many other kids might be playing there. Not long ago, on one of our visits to Chicago, I took you there, too, Ben. It was strange to see you climbing all over the equipment with your usual aplomb. I did not feel entirely comfortable at the sight. Forgive me, but I had the odd sensation that you were an intruder. Over the past thirty years, the playground had changed beyond recognition. The original swings and slides had been updated by park planners mindful of both the safety of the young and the litigiousness of the times: sturdy plastic had replaced dangerous metal, sharp edges had been rounded, seesaws had been omitted altogether. (Perils are mushrooming everywhere in the late twentieth century.) Face-lift or not, though, that park was still Hannah's and mine. We'd left our mark on it. So many stories made up there, the ground was inundated with our plots.

It was only three blocks from our houses, but that was faraway enough. Beyond the faraway park we never ventured, either to its continuation on the other side of the busy street called Asbury, where there were softball fields and tennis courts and an open area that was turned into a skating rink in the winter, or to the backyards and alleyways that spilled into the park at its outer limits, where the boundaries were ambiguous and one could hardly tell where the playground ended and private property began. (Dear Ben, I know *you* would have gone farther.) But Hannah and I were not tempted by the prospects of trespassing. We had plenty of other adventures to keep us occupied.

We would commandeer a large play structure set on wheels embedded in the sand, with a series of metal platforms and stepladders, that was probably supposed to resemble a fire truck. I would hop on one platform, Hannah on another a few feet below, and we would begin to spin our tale. We narrated to each other, Hannah taking her cue from me—I was the captain of the story, plotting its course, navigating it smoothly through climax to denouement, and Hannah was an expert first mate, who could sense from the tiniest change in inflection which direction I was likely to take, and could react in a split second to my every move. As we talked, we moved about the structure, climbing from one level to another as the scene changed, or, if the story called for it, leaping into the sand and rolling underneath the platforms, where the coolness and the swath of shadow created an instant change of tone and mood in our narration. Five yards away was a large benign oak tree we sometimes fled to if our story called for a forest scene, or if we simply needed to escape from the mounting tension of our tale. If we felt our inspiration flagging, we ran to the swings, and, pumping our legs, urging ourselves ever higher and higher, we swung and talked, sometimes extending our arms, holding on tight to the chains and leaning as far back as we could, narrating upside down. That almost always brought us to the point where we could continue or, if we were close enough, bring the story to a thrilling conclusion.

I chose the period, and the locale. "The story takes place," I would start, in hushed tones, "*over a hundred years ago.*" "We're on a wagon train going to California." Most of the stories were dominated by my passion for pioneers and the Western Expansion. Hannah did not seem to mind. Along the way, a young girl who looked a lot like me ("willowy, with green eyes") always died of tuberculosis and was buried halfway to the promised land. We both got choked up over this, but we never permitted ourselves to actually cry—we understood, without having to verbalize it, that crying would have prevented us from completing the story. We had to function as both player and audience, and this necessitated a sort of divided consciousness—as audience, we could not help but enjoy our story and become emotionally involved, but as performers we had to be ready, at a moment's notice, to put a halt to our tears, find the thread of the narrative, and climb back up onto the stage. We knew that as an audience our pleasure in the performance would be diminished if we could not fulfill our roles as players. We absorbed all these complexities smoothly, and never let them impede the progress of the tale, which we both also tacitly understood to be all-important—the progress itself more significant than what was being told. If we'd been a little older, thinking about such things would have stymied us, but at ten more things seem possible.

"There's a man, an older man with a gray beard," I begin. "His name is Pierce. He's a widower."

Hannah pitches in: "His wife died in childbirth."

"Yes! That's why he wants to make the difficult journey west, to escape from his sorrow. He wants to start a new life in California because there's nothing left for him in Missouri."

"He's silent, but not cruel," says Hannah. "He barely speaks unless it's necessary. He has a brooding look."

"Yes, that's good! A brooding look." We are silent a moment, admiring our handiwork. "Brooding" is one of our favorite adjectives and we try to work it in whenever possible. "Sometimes, when the rest of the troupe is gathered around the campfire at night, inside the circle of wagons, eating their meals and singing, Pierce becomes restless. He takes his rifle and walks to the edge of the wagon's circle, beyond the firelight, listening to the crickets on the prairie. He leans on his rifle and stares out into the east, from whence he came."

"From whence he came," whispers Hannah.

"He's thinking of—of—"

"Corinna," says Hannah. She is good with names.

"*Yes.* How she suffered, bleeding to death and in terrible pain . . . nobody could help her, not even the doctor . . . the darkness was torn apart by her screams . . . the whole floor of their cabin was covered with blood, he was slipping in it . . ."

"And the child was stillborn."

"A baby boy. He's left them both behind in Missouri, buried side by side in the field behind the cabin. Life holds nothing for him anymore . . ."

"Wait," says Hannah. She holds up a hand. Her sallow cheeks are suddenly flooded with color, a sure sign that a plot development is imminent. "He's *not* traveling alone. He's with . . . a girl named Amanda . . . she's a lot younger, about eighteen or nineteen . . . she's all alone in the world and before they left he . . ." She looks at me for approval then decides to strike out on her own: "He married her!"

"Hannah! That's good!" Hannah, bashful, ducks her head and tugs at her long ponytail, which is slung tidily across her left shoulder.

"But why did he marry her?" I ask a moment later. "If he wants to be alone? I mean, there was nothing left for him in life."

We come to a halt, faced with a narrative snarl. Then I say, "She's an orphan . . . she worked as a scullery maid for a family in town and they treated her badly . . . she wanted to go west to make a new life for herself and . . ."

Hannah says, "She can't go west all by herself . . . she's a woman alone . . . Pierce offers to marry her so that they can travel together. In exchange she'll cook for him, do the wash . . ."

I continue: "But the night before they are married, Pierce has a solemn talk with Amanda. He says to her, 'Amanda, I am very fond of you, but there is something I want you to understand. I can never love another woman again. I will always treat you with complete respect and I will help you as much as it is in my power to do so. But we will be man and wife in name only.'"

"'In name only,'" breathes Hannah.

"'I think of you as my daughter. Do you agree to this arrangement? Can you find it in your heart to marry without love, to a middle-aged man who is old enough to be your father?' Amanda lowers her eyes modestly. 'I agree, Pierce. I will go with you wherever you go.' Secretly she is in love with him. But she makes a vow to never let him know this . . . ever . . ."

"So their marriage is not—consummated?" asks Hannah, blushing.

"No. They sleep in separate beds. In the wagon."

There is always an Amanda in our stories: pale, modest, downtrodden, furtively intelligent, overlooked. This Amanda suffers nobly, in silence, while she is married to Pierce, respecting his need for solitude. She is his helpmate on the long arduous journey, feeding the oxen, making their meals of cornbread and beans, fetching water from the stream, mending the canvas roof of the wagon when it is torn. His respect for her grows. He treats her with gruff tenderness; slowly he becomes aware that his feelings for her have changed. Sometimes he finds himself staring at her for no reason at all. ("He wants to have sex with her?" says Hannah. "Of course," I reply.) Then, one night there is an Indian raid. The women and children huddle together while the men defend the camp. Many shots are fired; a few men die. When Pierce finally returns to Amanda, she forgets herself, throws her arms around his neck, cries, "Pierce! Pierce! Thank God you are alive!" Pierce begins to kiss her, first on the cheek, then on the neck, then their lips find each other . . .

"'At last I am truly your wife,'" says Hannah. I wanted to say that line myself, but I am generous, I give it to her.

After our stories, we would walk home slowly, two overheated ten-year-old girls cooling down, as spent and satisfied as our lovers. We were solemnly aware that we had pushed back the curtain from the universe a few more inches that day, revealed a sliver more, and then a sliver more again. All our stories were more or less the same: soft-focus erotica, tales of thwarted love and its ultimate reversal, sex. Sex was the portal through which we were destined to pass, we knew. The clinical details we had a handle on; but nobody, absolutely nobody, could tell us all the particular feelings we might experience when a man's penis penetrated our vaginas. So what we didn't know, we made up. We were generally pleased with our version of events.

Sometimes I went to Hannah's house after school to wait

until my mother came home from work. The kitchen where we would sit and do our homework smelled of kasha and old linoleum. There was always something dreary and glutinous cooking in a giant cast iron pot on the ancient stove, which had a pilot light that had to be lit by hand. Nobody ever opened any windows in that house. Occasionally, as we worked, Hannah's father would pass through the kitchen in his stocking feet, mumbling, inching slowly forward, taking an eternity to cross the ten feet between one hallway door and another. A powerful odor of unwashed socks would crowd out the porridge smell. We held our breath, pencils suspended, until he had gone.

I was supposed to call my mother before I left Hannah's, to make sure she was home. But I was terrified of using the telephone. The thought of speaking into a receiver, even to my mother, filled me with a chill fear. I did not know how to begin or end conversations, I did not know how to fill the emptiness resounding from the phone cables; I could no more casually pick up a phone than I could casually knock on a closed door. It was too unscripted; in my own stories I was in charge, but there was no telling what response I would solicit from behind the door, beyond the receiver. Most of the time Mrs. Krempel called home for me. But one day she'd had enough.

She folded her arms over her bosom and refused to dial. She was a formidable woman; wigless, as she often was around the house, her forehead was high where the hair had receded and the hair on her skull was sparse, showing great patches of whitish-gray scalp. She had warts on the backs of her hands. She crossed over to the extreme side of ugliness, which is fascinating, like beauty. I could never take my eyes off her when she was in the room.

She pointed to the phone. "Dial. You know your phone number?"

"Yes . . . but I . . ."

"A big girl like you should know how to use the phone. Dial."

I picked up the receiver, poked my index finger in the first hole. I felt sick to my stomach. I dragged my finger around the loop once, heart pounding. Then I hung up.

"Don't be nonsensical. There's nothing to be afraid of. It's just a telephone."

It took me three false starts to dial my complete number. Each time I begged her to dial for me. She shook her head. "I can wait all night."

The only reason I didn't cry was because I hated her so much: the hate dried up my tears.

Finally I managed to call home; I held the receiver close to but not touching my ear and heard it ringing. In a panic, I held it out to her.

"You're just stubborn. Your mother doesn't see that, but I do. She indulges you in your fears, like giving you too much candy. So you hang onto them."

Probably she was right. I *was* stubborn, most particularly about my fears, which I felt defined me in some way, and my mother *was* soft on me. Mrs. Krempel felt it was her duty to squelch these tendencies. It was a battle that was already weighted in her favor; when an adult goes to war with a child, the outcome is foreordained. She broke me, and after that I knew how to use the telephone, could reach for one anywhere and speak into it at will, as if it were the most natural thing in the world to be talking into a box, to an incorporeal voice which might be two miles away or two thousand.

"You see?" Mrs. Krempel was fond of saying to me, whenever I phoned home, "Isn't it better this way, now you can be more independent. You'll thank me some day." She put great stock in this, the assurance of my future gratitude.

In reality, I never once considered being grateful to her. It's a secret source of pleasure for me, knowing that I am *not* grateful to Mrs. Krempel, thus negating her expectations. She began to like me better now that I was more obedient and I believe she even believed *I* liked *her*. She was mistaken. I tolerated her; she was the price I had to pay for Hannah and the faraway park. But they were both worth it, always.

To my great regret, Ben, I lost sight of Hannah before adolescence. She was sent to a religious school and, as I heard through my parents, made an arranged marriage soon thereafter. Then, the submersion in a carefully circumscribed community, where even the route you must travel from home to synagogue on Shabbat is mapped out for you in advance. For an Orthodox Jew, little is left to chance: there is never any question about what to eat or read, when to grieve, make love, bathe, or pray. Even her hair would not be a worry: the ponytail would have been cut off in a ritual ceremony before her wedding, and from then on a wig would have served as fashion statement. How different from the way my life progressed, Ben, with all its waywardness, randomness, and sensuality. I began this piece by lamenting Hannah's disappearance, but now I see that perhaps she had an advantage over me. It was a community that more or less kept her safe, I guess, by leaving no room for risk. What would the Talmudic scholars have made of AIDS? In that marvelous and frustrating religion there are laws covering every aspect of life, and myriad interpretations of those laws. I imagine the learned men calling an emergency convention, putting their heads together—a sea of black *kipots,* if you were looking down from above!—and whispering in urgent Hebrew, trying to make sense of the epidemic. I enjoyed boundless freedom, compared to Hannah, whom I thought of pityingly as "poor

Hannah," when my thoughts happened to turn to her at all, which was not often. Now, ironically, my life is as circumscribed as hers: the same pills at the same time day in and day out; every three months, a blood draw and a visit to the specialist; every six months, the gynecologist; every year, a chest x-ray. I even have my own food restrictions: under no circumstances am I allowed to drink tap water, or consume sushi, Caesar salads, unpasteurized juices, steak Tartar, or raw oysters.

Wouldn't Hannah be surprised to learn that I really *did* emigrate to California? She would not be surprised, though, to learn that I still carry a torch for wagon trains, enough to drag my family on a vacation to eastern Oregon so that I could finally satisfy my desire to stand in a wagon rut. (You stood in the rut too, Ben, and faced the great valley countless pioneers had faced before you.) I would like Hannah to know what that felt like. She would have loved that grand sweep as much as I did—the green distances, the halo of mountains surrounding the valley, the oceanic sky. We could still share pleasure in that sight, even after the passage of time and in spite of our vastly divergent lives. Once, some meddlesome grownup asked Hannah what she wanted to be when she grew up. I heard her answer dutifully, "A nurse." But I knew she was lying. She wanted to be an astronaut, a Russian princess, a pirate. And still does, I'll bet.

Poetry

More than twenty years have passed since my fleeting friendship with Cal Epstein, but these two decades have not been enough to erase my shame and sense of failure. Cal Epstein is not his real name, of course. I would be mortified if the actual man were ever to discover that I still thought about him enough to make him the subject of an essay. Names must be changed to protect your innocent mother, Ben, who is a delicate organism, subject to fits of self-castigation and moodiness.

Cal was a high school poet who later became a poet in the outside world as well. In other words, he kept his desires intact and never lost sight of his gift. Whether he will become a famous poet is still unknown. But he published in reputable journals, got a Ph.D. from Harvard, and fulfilled many of the promises he made to himself (and to his admirers) when he was seventeen years old. I'd had a ferocious crush on him ever since our freshman year, but Cal had many advantages over me: for one thing, he had never been an adolescent. He seemed to have bypassed this stage and proceeded straight into the airy confidence of young manhood. So we rarely had any contact with each other—until we both ended up in a summer school creative writing course and an acting class in the summer before our senior year.

The classes were not remedial, but extracurricular. They were the sort of thing bright teenagers did with their spare time; we didn't go cruising in the malls or hang out at beaches. We were used to the routine of school and classes and we felt a bit lost without it. We didn't really know how to have fun. The biggest difference between Cal and me was that he hung out with kids who did know how to have fun, got invited to parties and dances and so forth. But they respected his inability to have fun without ridiculing him—he had a special talent for attracting people's notice and respect. I, on the other hand, was completely overlooked by the fun crowd. Cal could claim to be a part of this group, but superior to it, but I had few claims except anonymity and, perhaps, a certain ability to irritate people when I did manage to penetrate their field of vision.

I don't know if anybody except me found Cal to be good looking. Probably they did. He was short and a little rotund, with a round face and soft babyish cheeks, twinkling brown eyes, and a mass of light brown curly hair. He wore his hair a bit long, thinking of Shelley, no doubt. The long hair and his fair smooth skin—I don't remember him ever having any facial hair—gave him a rather effeminate appearance. But he had a decidedly masculine way of commanding people who came into his orbit, of orchestrating them. And his belief in his talent was enormous and infectious. I think the combination of his soft exterior and his sharp determined will was exciting to me, and to others.

Cal and I had all the right ingredients for a rich friendship. After all, we were both writers, and we were involved in many of the same activities. We took Advanced Placement courses in English, history, and French. Both of us wrote for the school newspaper, and both of us had pieces performed by the reader's theater. The school's literary magazine was rather more splashed with his poetry than it was with my prose, and there were more pictures of him in the yearbook, but aside from that we were equals in academic achievement. I often felt as if we were secret competitors, although I am quite certain he was blissfully unaware that he was competing with me. The fretting was all on my side. I envied him, which prevented me from acting in any way naturally around him—or, for that matter, from talking to him at all. I was often angry at him, feeling that *he* ought to envy *me*. And perhaps it was true, he did owe me some envy—as one talented student writer to another. But I did not know how to claim that envy, or to claim any of my rights as a bright young woman. I felt as if I had none, especially where Cal Epstein was concerned. We did all the same things in high school, our paths followed the same trajectory, and yet he was beloved by so many, and I was ignored by so many. And so any attempts he or I made at friendship were quickly aborted.

So, that summer, I felt as if I had been offered my last chance when I discovered that Cal was in both of my classes. Next year we would both graduate; this summer, anything could happen. The braces were finally off my teeth—proof enough that the world was full of possibilities. And, whether because the strict social codes we obeyed during the school year were somewhat relaxed during the summer, or simply because there was no one else he recognized in the class, Cal was markedly friendly to me. I was flattered by the way he accepted me as an equal and more—as a fellow novitiate in the writing life, a devotee. He would beckon me to sit next to him when I entered the room, would turn to ask me questions during discussions. ("What do *you* think about that, Paula? Weren't you saying just yesterday you don't like the overuse of the present tense in so much contemporary writing?") We would walk out of class together, lingering to talk in the hallways before we separated for the hour between our writing class and our acting class. Of course I longed to spend this hour with him and often hoped that he might suggest we eat lunch together, but I never dared to suggest it myself. Still, our camaraderie was a settled thing, and I considered myself blessed to have that, at least. I admired the ease with which he fell into step with me, as if it were a perfectly natural thing for us to be friends. What was more, during our acting class, he clearly deferred to my superior talents and even, amazingly enough, asked my opinion about some of the scenes or monologues he had chosen to perform. He was no actor; he told me that he had signed up for the class in order to hone his elocution and performance skills. When the time came that he was publishing books and going on book tours and giving interviews and readings on radio and television, he

meant to be prepared. He implied that this time was imminent. I tried my best to be the earnest, beneficial critic he
seemed to crave.

But he was not nearly so deferential in our creative writing class. There he clearly reigned. His precocious gift for
poetry had attracted the attention of almost all the English
teachers, so the teacher in summer school was primed for
him and eagerly awaited his presence when she saw his
name on her class roster. She was always pointing out the
wonderful phrases, metaphors, and images in his poetry. She
instructed us to take note of his rhythms and rhyme schemes.
By the end of the first week all of us were thoroughly intimi-
dated and did not dare to offer anything more than the
blandest criticism, in a weak attempt to show that we were
still thinking for ourselves. The fact was, his poetry really
was wonderful and it was a body of work you could learn
from as a writer, even though he was only seventeen years
old. And it was truly a body of work—he wrote every day,
and experimented with different forms—lyrics, odes, free
verse. He was even working on a ten-book epic poem. I
think at his young age he had already mastered the discipline necessary to achieve anything as an artist, and that
must have accounted for his smooth absorption of adolescence. Who could not envy him? His path was so clear: all
he had to do was continue to refine his craft, assimilate experience and live passionately through his senses. That was
his job.

He was polite about his classmates' attempts, but exhibited a thinly disguised impatience when forced to hear too
much of them. When I read one of my short stories in class,
he was as usual very correct in his responses during the discussion afterward, but as we walked out the door together
he remarked, "Your work is conservative, isn't it?"

Conservative! Could any adjective be more disparaging than that! That word branded me. I understand now that while in one sense it is true—I have never been the sort of writer who experimented with form—in another equally valid sense, it is not true at all. Still, I took it so deeply to heart that it was months before I could write another word. It was the first time in my life that I'd ever had such a break in fluency—I'd always written reams upon thoughtless reams, enjoying it for its own sake and never stopping to judge myself. Now, after a single word from Cal, I had suddenly become self-conscious.

I smoldered; I plotted revenge. The next week in class, after Cal had read one of his poems out loud and the teacher looked at us in her bright expectant way and there was the usual cowed silence in the room, I summoned all the courage I had and spoke up.

"I'm, like, not really sure about this," I stammered. "But, ah, I think, you know, that metaphor about the flowers and then the one about the ship? In the fourth stanza? I think that's like, a kind of a mixed metaphor. I mean, I think you kind of start out with the flowers and then all of a sudden you're talking about ships . . . well, maybe that's okay, but . . . well, it seems sort of, well . . . maybe overdone? Or . . . or . . . weak or forced or something."

Cal himself did not respond; he knew it wasn't necessary for him to defend himself. That was the teacher's job. She jumped right in, explaining to me in great detail why I was wrong, deconstructing the metaphors for me, interpreting the images, lecturing on why the poem as a whole would suffer if that particular stanza was altered. Cal seemed pleased with her efforts. The other students remained ambivalent: on the one hand, they were in awe of my heroism, and on the other, they were inclined to believe she was right.

As we were filing out of the room, Cal took me by the arm and said, "I have an idea. We should get together between classes and discuss poetry. I don't know why I didn't think about it before. I know the perfect place—up in the theater, you know, there's that little lounge that no one uses? We could sit in there before acting class and no one would bother us, it's really private. Let's go up there now."

My heart was in my throat; I no longer had an urge for revenge. This was what I had hoped for—a lunchtime tryst. Even—or perhaps I should say *especially*—at the age of seventeen I knew what it meant when a boy invited you into a "little lounge" where you could be "private." I was mad with desire. I nodded, not trusting myself to speak.

The lounge was narrow, with one high window looking out on a courtyard. The largest item of furniture was a long divan, a sort of fainting couch, highly suited to a theatrical lounge. That took up most of the room, and then there was a table, and an armchair, and that was it. Upon entering the room, Cal immediately perched on the back of the armchair, his feet resting on the pillow. As for me, I teetered demurely on the edge of the divan, not daring to sit back too far, to relax. I kept my hands on my knees in readiness. It seemed to me that at any moment Cal might fly down off his perch and ravish me. I awaited that moment with devilish, swooning, calculating patience.

But as it turns out, I waited in vain. What he did was just what he had said he was going to do—discuss poetry. His poetry, in particular. The tryst was instructional, although the nature of the instruction was of course not what I had hoped. He read beautifully—his elocution studies had paid off. He had a piping, rather feminine voice, but his range of expression was powerful and he made up in confidence what he lacked in tonality. I am afraid I never listened to any of his poems because I was frantically trying to come up with something clever to say after he had finished reading. I sweated delicately in the close room. Somehow I always did manage to find something pertinent and intelligent to say, for all my panic—that was where my superior talent for acting stepped in and saved me. Cal usually looked pleased at my comments and once or twice he said to me, "I really like doing this. You're a sensitive reader. I mean, I feel like you come close to understanding what I'm trying to say."

He would elucidate the meaning of his poem, saying to me, "Now look at this one line. I think you should take a closer look at the alliteration . . ."

And I would scramble to make some pithy remark. And he would look at me appreciatively, cocking his head to one side and saying, "You're really getting this. You really are."

I was flattered, but I wanted to be groped and violated. I felt crude in comparison to ethereal Cal, perched high on his chair, his curls waving slightly in the breeze from the ventilator. My desires made me feel ashamed and guilty and hypocritical, like I was a traitor to poetry. Our lunchtime sessions went on for weeks and weeks. He clearly wasn't going to fuck me, and I was exhausted from the constant effort of trying to be original and witty—and for what was I exerting myself, after all? For nothing. For mere *talk*.

I told my girlfriends that Cal Epstein and I were meeting in a small room with a big couch three days a week, reading poetry together.

These fellow virgins looked impressed. But one of them, a girl I didn't trust, said, "I just hope he's not taking advantage of you."

It occurred to me that in a way he was using me, just not in the way that she had insinuated. I felt humiliated: somehow this was much worse than if he had been bragging about his conquest to the whole football team. *That* I wouldn't have minded.

Sexual innocence seemed to me then, as it seems to me now, a terrible handicap in human relationships. In a few short years, Ben, I would have known all too well how to topple Cal off his perch on the armchair and onto that magnificent and underutilized divan. (Strange, isn't it, that *virginity* was my problem then?) But, in life, enlightenment is almost always a little tardy. I did not understand Cal's hesitation, especially since I did everything I could to make myself such an easy target. Perhaps he was simply waiting for a signal from me, although I cannot believe he was blind to my adoration. Perhaps he was innocent himself. There was always the possibility, of course, that Cal was not interested in girls—at seventeen I was aware of such possibilities, although I had no idea that they might exist so close to home. I knew, though, that in the past Cal had had girlfriends. Later in life I learned that this is no proof of anything, but at that time I took it as solid evidence that I was at least heading in the right direction.

Since it was summer, instinct told me to wear pretty sundresses with bare shoulders and paint my toenails. I showed off my new straight teeth whenever possible. Yet these embellishments seemed to be antithetical to the nature of poetry discussion, and I felt, again, slightly hypocritical, but what else could I do? I understood in a vague way that some kind of crime was being perpetrated against me as a woman, and I resented it and rebelled by looking as attractive as I could.

But it all did no good, and Cal remained oblivious—feigned or otherwise—to my designs on him. Worse, he began to use me as a confidante, which is probably one of the most terrible insults a woman in love can ever receive from the object of her affections. He read me love poems he had written for a girl who was anorexic. I knew her: a sallow, morose female whom he had somehow invested, to my amazement, with vast poetic and romantic properties. What's so romantic about sticking your finger down your throat three times a day? I wanted to shout to him. Why don't you take me, I'm naturally thin and you should see what I can eat, double orders of French fries and hot fudge sundaes and I never gain an ounce.

Our relationship deteriorated to the point where he began to discuss politics with me, and it was then I gave up all efforts to try and impress him and began to flex my sense of humor instead. I'd always been funny, but I suppressed this quality with boys I liked because I thought it wasn't ladylike. Only homely girls were funny; none of the pretty ones you saw on television or the movies were ever funny. It was so depressing. But since I was absolutely invisible to Cal Epstein as a woman, what the hell? I'd let it all go. I discovered I could be ironic. This really *did* impress him, and once he said to me, after I had made some amusing remark, "You're great, Paula, you know that?" I felt I was making progress, until the day he commented about a girl in our acting class, "You know, she is the most beautiful girl I have ever seen in my entire life." She was the most beautiful girl I had ever seen in my entire life too: pale, pale skin, blond hair, great bones. And all this time I'd nurtured a small hope that perhaps he was simply above noticing the beauty of women, that his head was occupied with far loftier thoughts—perhaps that explained his indifference to my valiant show of skin, my flash of new teeth. My hopes were dashed.

And then the summer ended and it was time to go back to school. In retrospect, I see that my interlude with Cal Epstein enriched me as a human being; he was a terrific poet, and a good teacher, and a wonderful conversationalist. Later in life, as I have said, he became renowned for all these qualities, and so in some ways I was lucky to have the benefit of his undivided attention for at least those few weeks. But I did not see it that way at the age of seventeen. I saw that he had given me nothing I really wanted.

In that last year in high school he rejoined his former group, I rejoined mine. I do not think he consciously made a decision not to continue our friendship; I think the evolving patterns of our separate lives simply prevented us from continuing what we had started in summer school. We did have an Advanced Placement French class together; he sat up front, interjecting French remarks from time to time and trading French witticisms with the teacher, and I sat in the back, watching the back of his neck and seething with resentment because he never turned around to speak to *me*. French had never been my strong point. I could not show off here, so I had no weapons.

After we went to college I wrote him an embarrassing and incriminating letter, excerpted here:

Dear Cal,

Congratulations on getting into Harvard. It must be wonderful to attend a school where everybody is your intellectual equal. Of course, there were some people in high school you deigned to talk to, deeming them to have sufficient cerebral capacity for your purposes. I suppose, for a while, I was one of those people . . .

. . . I wonder if you remember that I write also? I believe I might have mentioned it. (In the creative writing class we took together that summer, I didn't get to read my stories very often as so much of the class time was taken up with a discussion of your epic poem, "Badges of Honor.") I doubt you recall even one paragraph of my stories. You never said much about them. I, on the other hand, offered whole dissertations about your work . . .

It went on in this vein for awhile, then veered into a slightly more tremulous tone. (Here, Ben, I am afraid to say, your mother often echoes Eeyore, one of your favorite characters from *Winnie-the-Pooh*.)

> I know you have many more valuable friends now but perhaps the memory of the time we spent together still has some meaning for you. Perhaps not. In any case, in the name of friendship, would you mind if I ventured just a few more parting comments? (After all, we never had a chance to say goodbye. You were far too busy saying goodbye to other people; why should you bother with me?) You must believe that what I say is spoken in the spirit of honesty and integrity. I *care* about what happens to you, as a poet and a human being. That's why I'm writing this.
>
> I never got a chance to tell you this, because you were so busy praising yourself all the time, but I think a lot of your poetry is mediocre. Your meter is sloppy and your rhymes are off (sometimes). And you're too fond of making yourself deliberately obscure. I *know* you had some of your teachers fooled. But you didn't fool me! . . .

At this point the letter began to disintegrate alarmingly:

> You probably don't even like getting advice from such a nobody. You are probably just laughing at this letter and saying I'm jealous. Well, I pity you. Someday we might meet at a literary party in New York and I might not even remember you . . .

He wisely never answered. No doubt this was a love letter, but the sender did not know herself well enough to recognize it as such. And she was too proud to write without dissembling, which made this a very shameful letter indeed. Let your mother's experience be a lesson to you, Ben. If you are ever about to commit your love to paper—and by all means be aware of the dangers inherent in this decision and proceed with caution—be sure that you offer an honest expression of it. Otherwise your attempt is bound to fail. Cal could only have been amused and gratified after receiving that letter—not the reaction I had hoped for at all.

Years later when I was already married and living in San Francisco, I read in the small print of the literary section of the weekend paper that Cal was going to be giving a poetry reading in Berkeley. So I went, and sat in the back, and watched him read. He looked the same as ever: pale, chubby cheeks, the curls, the feminine voice. The poems were ones I had read not too long ago in the *Paris Review*. They were brilliant. The audience stood up and clapped after he had finished. He had an appealing gentleness, a humility, that I did not remember him having in high school. Perhaps, as I had taught myself so painfully to be confident, he had taught himself to be humble. We were both the same people we had been twenty years earlier, only we had refined our characters and learned how to live in the world. We were both survivors, too—we both still wrote.

But if you imagine that after his reading I joined the crowd of well-wishers clustering around him, thrust out my hand, reintroduced myself, and suggested we talk over a cup of espresso at a nearby Peet's coffeehouse, then you would be wrong, Ben, and I would have to accuse you of not paying attention so far. I let him go and lost my chance. Maybe I was afraid he would remember that awful letter. But there was an even worse possibility—maybe he would not remember me at all. That was unbearable. Anybody would have slunk away, wouldn't they? Yet in spite of this incident I retain a stubborn faith in the dogged forward advance of my beleaguered self-esteem. And these days I am bolder—having faced death, surely I can face the polite, blank stare of a former high school crush. If in another twenty years I am offered another chance to renew my acquaintance with Cal Epstein, surely this time I will take it? What do you think?

Silence

Ben, you know me as a woman with a voice, and it might be hard for you to imagine that I ever lacked one. I speak out to policymakers and politicians; I tell my tale freely and comfortably to teenagers who need to hear it. I talk to strangers on the phone about sex. There have even been times in my life when I have spoken far too much—when my voice has wounded or bored people, because I did not know when to stop.

But at the age of seventeen, I spoke too little. This affliction was so acute that I wonder if people suspected I was deaf and dumb, or mentally disabled, or simply rude. Most of my teachers found this trait to be insupportable. I was terrified of speaking out in class; the consequences of raising my hand to be called on—having to answer a question or make a comment—seemed too terrible to risk. I certainly had comments to make. I had read everything and I had always done my homework. That was not the problem. My teachers could not understand why there should be such a discrepancy between my written work in class and my "oral presentation," as they called it. I contributed nothing to class discussions. Some teachers were belligerent and called on me anyway, just to spite me: I believe they enjoyed watching me squirm and blush. Others had individual conferences with me in which they threatened to lower my overall grade by a certain percentage if I did not offer at least a specific number of comments each class period. (I used to wonder, what exactly constituted a comment? How many words did it have to contain, or how many minutes did it have to consume? And just how far apart did these comments have to be? I could not get the answers to these questions, however, because I did not dare to ask them.) One teacher sent me to a guidance counselor. But nothing could deter me from my stubborn shyness. I would far rather have had my grade point average drop than speak up in class.

There was only one teacher in high school who really understood me and accepted me the way I was. He was my Advanced Placement English teacher in my senior year, and his name was Mr. Garrity. I immediately experienced a deep feeling of communion with him, when he opened up *Gone with the Wind*, read us the first sentence, and declared to us, "By the end of this year, each of you will understand why *Gone with the Wind* is an excellent story but not a work of art. You will be able to distinguish between a good book and a great one." I had done enough reading to sense these things intuitively: I knew that there was goodness and greatness, that some books were literature and some were not. My ideas about what constituted greatness were unformed, incomplete, but my convictions about the whole subject of books in general were tough and passionate. This man, this Mr. Garrity, he was the real thing. Ben, always trust yourself at seventeen to recognize what's genuine and what's not. Later in life, you may not be so sure.

The reading list was a rich brew—*Mrs. Dalloway* and *The Brothers Karamazov, Julius Caesar, Hamlet. The Death of Ivan Ilych* and short stories by Chekhov. Shakespeare's sonnets. The tragedies of Aeschylus. Poems by Matthew Arnold and Robert Browning and Wallace Stevens and Wordsworth. It had variety, and rhythm, and heft. It refused to capitulate to the standard notion that adolescents were creatures stymied by wildly fluctuating hormones and demanding social schedules. It took no account of after-school swimming practice or dating jitters or even college applications. It ploughed right through those things and took us, Mr. Garrity's Advanced Placement English class, along with it.

We were expected to write intelligently about everything we read. Mr. Garrity assumed—mostly correctly, in our case—that we had been well-trained in the skill of essay writing during our first three years of high school. The five-paragraph paper, with its introduction, three supporting paragraphs, and conclusion, had become a part of our consciousness. We knew about topic sentences and transitional phrases and such things. The more sophisticated among us knew to avoid the adverbs "firstly," "secondly," and "thirdly," and how to make graceful use of the wonderful word "nonetheless." It was Mr. Garrity's intention, however, to take us above and beyond these earthbound, adolescent rules, to let us soar. His assignments were imaginative—to teach us about the limitations and restrictions of genre fiction, he instructed us to read a series of genre books (the genre we chose was up to us) and write a paper dissecting them; to learn about research techniques, he had us look up old crimes on microfiche in the public library and then reconstruct the tale as best we could, like a detective, using different sources; to learn about stream-of-consciousness, we were required to write a short story in the manner of *Mrs. Dalloway;* to learn about meter, he ordered us to write a sonnet. We were taught to recognize dramatic irony and the always tragic character flaw called hubris. He organized a field trip for us to see the *Barber of Seville* at Chicago's Lyric Opera, and he regularly had speakers visit our classroom, including a well-known writer of juvenile fiction. He encouraged us to read the newspapers and had us keep clippings and write brief comments about them in a journal. In short, he was one of the finest teachers I have ever had, with a boundless generosity, and a noble, spirited demeanor. Ben, my wish for you is that every one of your teachers will be remarkable, that you will never run across a dullard or a prig to sour your school days. Yet even if you have only one Mr. Garrity in your life, I will consider you to be lucky.

Much as I loved this man, I could not speak in front of him. I could not gratify him—or myself—by forming a cogent comment in class. I wanted to badly enough. I wanted to present him with a gift of my thoughts, spoken in my voice and in my words. I was terrified, though, that my ideas would be rendered unintelligible in the translation from thinking to speaking, or, worse, that they would be construed as mundane. I could not risk such a misunderstanding. In class discussions, which were always energetic and avid, some other, more articulate student would always beat me to the punch and say exactly what I wanted to say. And I did not have the verbal sophistication or the elocutionary skills to elaborate on someone else's comment; I wanted to be the *first* to come up with an idea, not the second. It would have been mortifying to me to appear to be parroting someone else's words. Phyllis would have been puzzled by me now, so different from the show-offy little girl she'd known.

Sometimes during one of these discussions, I would become aware of Mr. Garrity's eyes upon me. He knew; he recognized my struggles. He would nod ever so slightly, and a faint warmth radiated from his alabaster skin, a warmth he seemed to be directing at me, the way someone would hand you a scarf to wrap yourself in on a chilly day.

Say it, I would urge myself. Just spit it out. But I was mute; I could not accept the scarf that was offered to me. Mr.

Garrity averted his face, so as not to witness my profound embarrassment.

Because I could not speak, I wrote beautifully for Mr. Garrity. He brought out the best in me. I wrote calmly, but with elation, in a state of grace, and each sentence appeared as a clear, gleaming, perfectly cut jewel in my mind the moment before I committed it to paper. There was little struggle involved—I imagined this was the way the prophets spoke, the voice of God rollicking through them, hollowing them out, flattening all else in its path. And I loved every word, the way God loved every creature in his dominion. I treated even the humblest articles and prepositions as if they were worth a king's ransom in gold.

Mr. Garrity returned my papers to me, not with words scribbled on the bottom of the last page, but with notes clipped to the top, typed flawlessly on good quality blue or gray stationery. "Your paper was a pleasure to read," he would write, or, "As usual, I was delighted to be privy to your insights and discoveries . . ." He praised my style, and occasionally gave me advice for improving it further. He touched upon all the salient points of my papers, lauded my original thinking and told me he learned new things about books that had been long familiar to him, by seeing them through my eyes. He would not tolerate grammatical and spelling mistakes and he made it clear that I was far too good a writer to allow my work to suffer from such blemishes: however, he also made it clear that he regarded perfect grammar in itself as a rather minor virtue, akin to neat handwriting and organized index cards. He focused his eyes, and mine, on more Olympian heights. When I wrote the stream-of-consciousness story for him, he wrote back, "This work is publishable. Have you thought about sending it away to a magazine?" What was wonderful about these notes was that he did not feel he had to temper his passion by manufacturing criticisms when he had none. He did not feel compelled to be professorial. He simply allowed himself to be joyful, without restraint.

These were love notes, I guess, the way my papers themselves were engendered from love. In fact that whole year we carried out a kind of love affair, right under everybody's noses, without arousing the least suspicion. But it was the most purely cerebral love affair I have ever engaged in, and perhaps the most memorable. We never exchanged glances, although I always sat up front; I was always careful to look to a space just to the right or left of him, and he, the soul of delicacy, always looked over my head when he asked a question in class. To all apparent purposes we were indifferent to one another. There were no teacher-student conferences, no flirty hellos or bye-byes. I never asked him to explain an assignment to me (the idea seemed laughable; I always knew instinctively what he wanted; I absorbed his assignments whole, took them deep into myself), and I never asked for his advice about choosing a topic. I never, God help me, discussed books or poems with him—I wouldn't have known how to begin. I was not part of the chatty contingent of students who gathered around his desk before class started and after class had ended, laughing and joking with him. To see him holding court you would have supposed that he had several favorites, and you would never have counted me among them. I marveled at my classmates who had this relationship with him, but I was not jealous. I knew exactly what I meant to him.

I can remember only two occasions when we spoke. The first time was to request a favor. Carol Blumberg and I were in another class together and we were working on a tough project that happened to be due on the same day as one of Mr. Garrity's assignments. She urged me to ask for an extension for both of us; somehow she sensed that he would be more amenable to a request coming from me. So, stumbling, blushing, I approached him and said, "Mr. Garrity, I wonder if you could grant an extension on this paper for Carol and I."

He tucked his rather pointy chin into his chest and frowned. "'Carol and me,'" he replied. "'Carol and I' would be a correct phrase if you were using it as the subject of the sentence, but you were using it as the object. And, yes, you may have an extension until Tuesday."

You can be sure I never made such an error again.

The other occasion was near the beginning of the fall semester, after he had first become acquainted with my work. He asked me to stay a few minutes after class. When all the others had left, he turned to me and said, "I want you to know, you don't ever have to speak up in class if you don't want to."

I was stunned. I waited for the inevitable "but" that I knew from experience must follow. There was no "but." There were no questions or prying. He didn't ask me if things were all right at home, as one teacher had.

He nodded and turned his back slightly, gathering the papers on his desk. That was really all. I had been dismissed.

He meant what he said; I don't think he intended it as bait to get me to open my mouth, to make me feel guilty or foolish. It was not a subtle threat. I think he understood that my silence was a part of who I was and that it could not be easily translated into articulation and eloquence. He accepted it, the way you had to accept things about people you loved; my silence had existed long before he had known me, and it would have been egotism on his part to believe that he could change me.

I took him at his word. I never did participate in class, not once. I never raised my hand and he never called on me.

Looking back I'm surprised that I did not feel the need to show off, because I was by nature a vain girl. (As Phyllis had surmised.) But my shyness canceled my vanity, I suppose: or the savage fidelity I had to my shyness. I never told anyone else in that class about the notes Mr. Garrity wrote to me or the secret pact of silence we had made. I'm sure that there is not a student in that class who would remember me now, not by a single gesture, or a smile, or a laugh. And certainly not by a word.

On the last day of class, Mr. Garrity had us do something that seemed to me at the time and still seems to me very beautiful. He unrolled a long spool of yarn and had us all hold onto a section of it, so that we were joined hand in hand by this circle of yarn. Then he read us a poem by Yeats:

> When you are old and grey and full of sleep,
> And nodding by the fire, take down this book,
> And slowly read, and dream of the soft look
> Your eyes had once, and of their shadows deep;
>
> How many loved your moments of glad grace,
> And loved your beauty with love false or true,
> But one man loved the pilgrim soul in you,
> And loved the sorrows of your changing face;

He did not read us the last verse, which was incomparably sad:

> And bending down beside the glowing bars,
> Murmur, a little sadly, how Love fled
> And paced upon the mountains overhead
> And hid his face amid a crowd of stars.

This he knew we would learn soon enough in life; we did not need to hear it just yet.

He wanted us to know that he was the man who loved the pilgrim soul in us. After he read this, we were all perfectly still. I was holding my breath. Then he walked around the room with a pair of scissors and cut the yarn so that we were each left with a piece in our hands.

"Save that," he instructed us. "And whenever you look at it, think of the year we shared, and remind yourselves that we are still connected, through all we've read and discussed and written together."

The room exploded in applause. I took Mr. Garrity at his word and I saved the yarn, and all the notes he had written me, pasting them in a scrapbook. And now that I am older and grayer, I understand even more clearly the value of this gesture.

Mr. Garrity cleared paths for me. He showed me the way my passion lay—made me square my shoulders and face it, actually. Perhaps that is why I was so silent, all that year, because there was another voice I was trying so desperately to listen to. If I was not a writer, I was nobody. I could not be a lawyer or a doctor or an insurance agent. I had to become who I was and not anybody else, and that becoming, Mr. Garrity implied to me, was often a very difficult undertaking indeed. One needed moral fiber and great faith, the faith of heroes and revolutionaries. But he seemed confident that I would grow into myself, in time.

In the last note he wrote to me, he said, "You have talent far beyond that of a talented high school student. Write to me and let me know how you are doing."

But I did not write to him. Not the next year, or the year after that, or the year after that. I could not bring myself to—it is one of the great unsolved mysteries of my life. Was I afraid of the more personal relationship that letter writing might engender? Was I fearful that as an ordinary human being, and not a student, I would not quite measure up?

Letter writing to a former teacher was venturing into un-
charted terrain. But these reasons seem paltry, insufficient to
me, Ben, and I do not know what to make of myself, and my
alarming failure to hold onto Mr. Garrity, who of all people
in the world was certainly worth holding onto. It was carrying silence too far, to the point of fanaticism. You will remember that I turned back at the crucial point with Cal Epstein also, although in that case I did manage to write a
letter, albeit an unsolicited one. I abdicated my place in Mr.
Garrity's consciousness. He taught for many years and he
had hundreds of students and probably there were scores
among those whom he did keep in touch with and who remained figures of lively interest for him.

But I don't think he forgot me completely. This is the way
I like to imagine it, in my idealized version of events: that
the memory of me did not disappear altogether but broke
up into a thousand different fragments, lodged at random
throughout his body. Sometimes one of the fragments will
cause a small precise ache, which puzzles him. He cannot
locate its origin, and perhaps he attributes it to the vagaries
of aging. Each time the pain fades away again, he is a little
bit sad, and that puzzles him also. Then the sadness fades
too, and he returns to the vigorous, always engaging pursuits of his everyday life.

Astray

When I was twenty-three years old, I was hired as a Junior
Copy Writer for a small advertising agency specializing in
direct mail on Chicago's Michigan Avenue. At least, that
was the job I had been promised, but I was not there a week
before I discovered that I had really been hired as a secre-
tary. Something had gone seriously awry in my life. I felt

like someone who has been on a merry-go-round, gets off, and does not know what direction she is stumbling toward. Instead of easing up, the dizziness only got worse the more I struggled to right myself.

I typed drafts, charts, and letters at a madcap pace; my speed was ninety words per minute. If you will remember from a previous tale, Ben, at the tender age of eleven, I had taught myself to type. If I had ever dreamed then that my typing skills—which I believed then, in my innocence, had been nothing less than a gift from the gods—would have led me down such dreary paths, I would have taken a hammer to my beloved typewriter and smashed it beyond recognition. At some point in your life, Ben—all too soon, alas!— you will be hearing about something called "marketable skills." You are to avoid these at all costs. I am proud, as a parent, to be able to pass along this wisdom to you.

After two weeks I worked up the nerve to mention to Jim, the man who had hired me, that I was not actually *writing* any copy, just typing up what others had written. He replied that it was always wise to learn the business from the bottom up, and that he expected me to be writing copy soon. How soon? I asked, standing against his desk, so close I could finger his leatherbound pencil holder. I was aware this made him nervous. He smiled, shifted slightly in his chair so that we were no longer facing each other directly. He was about thirty-five years old, with sandy, receding hair, a long, lean face and a vapid, toothy smile. "You have to be ready to do that kind of work." Then he regaled me with a long, tiresome story about how he himself had started in the mail room, and now look who he was: an Assistant Executive Director.

I recognized this as a morality tale, and not a very clever one. I did not appreciate the transparent motive behind it— the desire to reeducate me. But I did understand that the tale itself was not as important as the fact that he had spent so much time in telling it that I would have no time left to say what I needed to. He had expertly circumvented me. It was a technique he had perfected and that he would use again in future encounters, and, prepared as I was, I was never quite able to maneuver myself into a position to speak my mind. He looked at his watch, and said, "Almost time for our company meeting. We'd better get going." We were forever having company meetings at this place. But I was desperate, so I plunged in. "But I already know how to write. I was an English major. I went to—" Jim put up a hand and said, "Yes, we know all about your academic successes. That's why we hired you. Because you are a very bright young woman with a lot of potential. But copy writing is a whole different ball game than that college stuff you've been doing. Believe me, it's not something you even want to rush into." He smiled, showing all his teeth. "We want to give you as much time as you need to learn." He stood up and moved toward the door. I opened up my mouth to speak again, but he patted me on the arm and said, "I'm so glad we had this conversation. It's always gratifying when my fellow workers feel they can open up to me." And in a flash he was gone.

Jim was right, Ben: advertising *was* a whole different ball game than that "college stuff."

It had been only a year and a half since I had graduated summa cum laude from Brandeis University with a degree in English literature. A resident poet and a visiting fiction writer both praised my writing highly; the visiting writer inscribed a copy of his book to me—"To a colleague from whom I have learned much and expect more." The poet strode down the aisle toward me in a crowded lecture hall—heads turning to see where he was going—stopped at my desk, and handed me a sheaf of papers, the short stories of mine he had read. He nodded his head and said simply, "You are a writer." It was the highest praise, immobilizing. For the longest time I could not get past that; I could not write anything else, for fear that what I wrote would demote me, that my subsequent work would prove me not to be a writer, or a colleague, or anything except simply a frightened girl. A certain kind of paralysis, Ben, or willful withdrawal, has always been my curse in life, and I pray that you are not similarly cursed. Now, though, circumstances have forced me to become a woman of action. I can no longer afford the time consumed by such perilous introspection. For economy's sake, I've learned to overtake myself.

All my professors expected me to go on to graduate school, but I resisted at first. I decided I wanted to try my hand in the "real world," although I had no idea what I meant by this, and I still don't. So I ran away from my teachers' expectations; after college I had a series of foolish jobs, then I went to Europe for the usual jaunt, and when I came back I took the job at the advertising agency. During all this time I had not written a thing. I had failed everybody. Not only had I not published the novel everybody had expected me to write, I had not even started it yet; I was not brushing shoulders with other literati at a New York coffee house, I did not write book reviews or go to book parties, I was not being solicited by editors who wanted me to promise my next three books to their publishing house. Everything I tried to write was bad, dishonest, self-indulgent, and dull, and I tore it all up. I was ashamed of myself for having let my teachers down. (Among these, of course, I included Mr. Garrity.) Would they ever trust another student again? Where would they find the energy to encourage another bright young English major, knowing that all their hopes for me had turned to dust? When I thought of my failures, I was remorseful not so much because I had ruined my own life, but because I had turned my dear teachers into cynics.

Yet I was determined to salvage something. I reasoned that if I could not be a famous literary light, then I would at least try to put some of my writing talent to use in another arena. The advertising agency seemed the perfect place to begin. It was practical, and yet there was scope for the imagination too. It was, let's face it, glamorous. Everybody wanted to work in advertising. It was an honest and lucrative profession: it would help me piece together my life again: I actually saw it as a sort of refuge from literature. Anything would have been, in truth. But instead of telling people I met that I was a writer, a statement that always engendered confusion and, worse, a lot of stupid questions about publications and romance novels (such as, "What kind of stuff do you write? Do you mean, like, romance novels?"), I could tell people, "I'm a copy writer," and they would understand instantly what I meant. It would be so comforting to have that qualifying adjective to bolster the noun. That alone seemed worth the effort. So I took the job. This was 1983 and everybody was making money, and I thought, why not me too? I'll be a careerist.

I was prepared for plenty of venality, because I'd heard a lot of stories about advertising agencies. But I was not prepared for banality. In addition to the one boss, Jim, I had another boss, Bill, who was short and squat and had adapted a loud jovial style to make up for his physical deficiencies. The two of them had founded the agency together and were eagerly jockeying for accounts and clients. They both had MBAs (from third-rate schools, I had noted) and they had each taken management training courses that taught them that the best way of managing people was to pretend to include them in all of the decision making in the company, so that they would be gratified and would feel as if they were actually working for *themselves* and not for Jim and Bill. I puzzled over their insistence on a sham democracy; at first I found it merely irritating and then, as time passed, increasingly insidious. In fact, Jim and Bill's mania for conformity soon began to smell more like communism than democracy. I thought this a wonderful joke on a profession that had its roots in unregenerate capitalism. These were dangerous times for me. One night when I had stayed until eight typing and retyping a difficult chart that Jim and Bill kept changing, which had complicated decimal points that were nearly impossible to align properly on the IBM Selectric, I was reprimanded by Jim, only half-playfully, for not smiling while I typed. "You know," he said to me, "this company belongs to you too. By typing this chart, you are helping to capture this account. What you're doing is just as important as what I'm doing. We're all in this together." I was horrified that he could lump me together with people like himself and Bill. I'm not like you at all! I wanted to cry. Oh God, could it really be true that my contribution to the world would take the form of an expertly typed six-column chart? I gritted my teeth and thought, "You horrible man, you can make a lot of noise about pretending to believe that I am as important as you, but I will never, never be convinced, if eons passed, that *you* are even one-sixteenth as important as *me*." And I made a point of not smiling for the next three days.

At one of our mandatory once a week agency meetings, Bill, the joker, put a paper cup on my head, laughed, and said I must wear my dunce cap. Their corporate strategy in general involved slashing everyone down to the lowest common denominator; there was an extremely beautiful Chinese woman, a graphic artist, and they told her she had to wear a bag over her face during meetings. We had to laugh because if we didn't it meant we were not all in sync. And it was very dangerous not to be in sync. We all came to dread these company meetings, which were interminable, vacuous, and deadly. I particularly dreaded the days when I was asked to take minutes (in the spirit of collectivism, we all took turns) because, try as I might, I never could understand what exactly was being discussed. At the following week's meeting, my minutes would be found lacking, and Jim and Bill would be sure to use this as yet another example of how my academic skills ("Didn't you have to take a lot of notes in those English courses?") could not hold water in the corporate world. Sometimes we played games designed to make us all feel more comfortable with each other. For example, we had to interview another person at the table and ask about their five favorite foods. Then we had to stand up and present a little speech about the person to the rest of the group. When it was my turn, I told my interviewer that I liked monkey's head, deep-fried rattlesnake meat, tuna fish stuffed okra, raw whale blubber, and dog steak. (You will recall, Ben, that even at the age of eight in Miss Higgins' class, I was already adept at offering unorthodox interpretations of class assignments.) Everybody laughed, including Bill and Jim, but afterward Jim took me aside and gave me a lecture about taking the games seriously. Humor had its place, but it was not productive to hide behind it; we were supposed to offer our "true thoughts" to one another. But of course I knew that I was not really expected to offer any of my true thoughts. I was just a platitude to them; so was the beautiful Chinese artist.

Every day I devised a new way of irritating Jim and Bill. I took to wearing my gold Phi Beta Kappa key around my neck to work. During meetings or when called in to talk to one of my bosses, I would dangle it idly between my fingers. The handwritten drafts Jim gave me were riddled with spelling errors; I would type up the draft, and return the original to him with red circles around his mistakes. Sometimes I put exclamation points. His syntax and grammar were equally awful but I resisted the temptation to rewrite anything because I knew he would pass it off as his own and be very pleased with himself, and I did not want to give myself any extra work.

I was beginning to understand that I would never be a Career Woman; no, not if my life depended on it. But I had just moved out of my parents' place, I had an apartment of my own, and I knew that I had to stay employed, at least for the time being. So I made the best of things I could. I turned to men and sex.

For you see, Ben, I had discovered Rapunzel's secret. Do you recall the fairy tale maiden who is locked up in a tower but lets down her long hair to the suitor who offers the correct chant? He is then able to climb up her hair to claim her and rescue her from a life of captivity. My captivity—in my own self, and within the prison of intellect—often felt to me as profound as Rapunzel's in her hated tower. Her hair is her connection to the world; ultimately, it provides the means of her escape. I took my cue from that ingenious damsel, but unlike Rapunzel, my forays outside the tower were only temporary. Sometime around the age of eighteen or nineteen I learned that I could get in or out at will. I did not want, necessarily, to stay out. I merely wanted a passport, and I found a convenient one. I let down my hair and rolled it up and let it down again, just as I pleased. I delighted in my newfound powers; and as I grew more accustomed to them, exercised them more often. Looking back, Ben, I can see that my often improvisational sex life was yet another manifestation of my love of a good story—I was not so far removed as I imagined from the little girl who used to spin wagon-train yarns in the faraway park. Only

now, of course, the story was overtly about me, and it was
acted upon the stage of my own life. All this was quite
thrilling. But I had confused myself with a fictional character, and that proved to be a fatal mistake.

I started a clandestine affair with our fifty-seven-year-old
creative director, a charming and degenerate alcoholic. I
was also dating a young graphic illustrator who had an office across the hall from ours; I flirted with him assiduously
at the elevators, until one day he asked me out to lunch.
There was also a Greek boy I saw occasionally, who was
the nephew of the Greek Orthodox Bishop of Chicago. The
Bishop lived in an elegant mansion on Chicago's Gold
Coast, and he was offering my boyfriend safe harbor, because he had run away from the draft in Greece. The Greek
used to borrow the Bishop's Lincoln Continental to take
me out on dates; when he knew that the Bishop was traveling for a few days on church business, he would sneak me
into the mansion and up to his well-appointed living quar-
ters. We would have sex, then go down to the black and
white tiled kitchen and eat some of the moussaka prepared
by the cook. (The Greek was generally petted and spoiled
by all the servants; he had grown a round belly from all the
food he'd been eating in America.)

Then there was my on-again-off-again Iranian-Jewish
boyfriend, a student, whose father had been a member of
the Shah's parliament before the disastrous events of
1979–1980. They had been wealthy in Iran, but in Chicago
the father was unable to find a job, and he was forced to sell
three fabulous rugs—the only valuables they had been able
to smuggle out of Iran—and with the proceeds bought a
small Laundromat, which supported them now. My boyfriend had accepted his fate; once in Chicago, he methodically set about learning English, and quickly became fluent.
Then he enrolled at the Illinois Institute of Technology,

where he was studying to be an architect. He was the least spoiled and the most pragmatic of his siblings, who all had problems in America. I had known him for two years and had not yet fallen in love with him, although I had tried to. Occasionally I slept with him to see if this would help but it never did.

Of all my boyfriends, he was the only one who truly loved me. If I was feeling blue, he would squeeze my hand and say, "Well, the first thing we have to do is get you happy again." My mother strongly intimated that I ought to "cultivate" my relationship with him. But there was something about him that irritated me—his pomposity, his dry humorless style, his fussy neatness, the frizzy black hairs on top of his head. He was exactly my age but he acted as if he were thirty-five years old—that's what serious emigration and a fall from grace will do for you. Sexually he was quite potent, which surprised me, but did not really convince me that I ought to settle for him.

Perhaps, Ben, this man could have saved me from the advertising agency, but I resisted being rescued. There was something else out there for me, I knew—not necessarily a man. Something waiting for me, and my Iranian-Jewish lover might prevent me from making this all-important rendezvous if I married him. I was intentionally cruel to him—somehow he activated my latent wickedness. I spent our dates talking about my other lovers, under the guise of needing a confidante. When he was visiting me, I would talk for a half hour on the phone with another man while he sat and read a magazine. He informed me that he would expect his wife to stay home and raise the children. I told him that I intended never to marry because I wanted to devote my life to writing. He told me that writing was fine for a hobby; a woman needed a hobby. I gave out my phone number to other men I met at parties he took me to. He remained stoic under every assault. He never complimented me on my looks, and I teased him about this. All the others told me I was beautiful in every second sentence. "Come on," I'd say, "you've got to admit I've got gorgeous legs. Just say it. What's the big deal?" His face turned to stone. He said to me, "If I were still living in my country, the wealthiest and most beautiful women would be lining up to marry me. I would have my pick and choose." I hated him.

I made a mental note to enjoy this time in my life, because I knew my career as a cavalier young woman was finite; the day would come when I would be forced to address myself to more serious topics. But at the moment, having plenty of lovers was just the antidote to the horrible advertising agency and all the puzzling questions as to what I was doing there and how in the world I would get out. So many dates—at least four nights out of the week— kept me well-separated from myself. And it was, of course, myself I did not want to meet. My behavior was not so unusual. In the early eighties, it was still possible to be light-hearted about sex. You were allowed to be driven about making money, but with sex it was best to keep a light touch.

Of my four established lovers, I was most seriously involved with the fifty-seven-year-old creative director and the young graphic illustrator. It was exciting, knowing I had two men who were just across the hall from one another. It began abruptly with the creative director: in a rebellious mood, I left our annual Christmas party and went straight to bed with him. His name was Alex, and he had been lured away at fantastic expense from an agency in Boston. He was supposed to be a wizard, a magic-maker. Jim and Bill danced and groveled before him. He possessed a depth of charisma that was unsullied by lots of bad behavior, such as coming back drunk from a two-hour lunch with a client, sauntering into the office at noon, taking impromptu three-day vacations. And fucking me. But of course, Jim and Bill did not suspect that he was fucking me, because they did not have enough imagination to conceive of the idea that a girl my age might find Alex attractive. That was one of the things Alex and I laughed about when we were alone together. He loved to make fun of Jim and Bill, of how stupid and gullible they were, of how he had tricked them into offering him a salary three times what he was worth at any agency in New York or Boston. He egged me on in my attempts to subvert the two Assistant Executive Directors. "You say yes to them too much," he advised me. "Just start saying no. For example, if they ask you to take their phone messages while they're at lunch, tell them you have better things to do. Or if they ask you to type up another memo about not wasting paper, tell them *that's* a waste of paper!" Sometimes I took his advice, sometimes I didn't. I did notice that no matter how much he mocked Jim and Bill, he always delivered for them. He had a way with clients; within a few months of his inauguration as creative director, we had five solid new accounts.

I suppose that in a half-hearted way I did hope that Alex might be of some use in my now rather unfocused objective to become a Junior Copy Writer. He did promise that he would help me, although, to my surprise, he uttered the same disclaimer that Jim and Bill had used—"when you're ready." I saw him about once a week, except for the times when his long-standing mistress, a woman closer to his own age, would fly to Chicago to visit him. He would take me out to expensive restaurants; the meal was always preceded by a tedious session of drinking at the restaurant's bar. I was not a big drinker; the first time I ordered Scotch and water (because I imagined this was what one ordered in the kind of restaurant that was paneled in dark wood and had brass rails at the bar), he winced and corrected me: "Say *Dewar's* and *ice*." I was young and had a healthy appetite and I would try not to let my stomach growl, while he slowly and methodically downed four highballs before dinner. I nursed my Dewar's and filled up on pretzels and hoped he would not notice that I was still on my first drink. But he was so drunk by the time we sat down at the table he assumed I was drunk too, which suited him. Then it would be his turn to wait while I ate ravenously; like most alcoholics, he consumed little solid food, and he was amused that I could eat so much. Sometimes he became impatient with me and said, "You already had enough bread. It'll go to your thighs."

After dinner we went back to his place to talk and have sex. The talk took place all around and during the sex; he was a great orator, a monologist. He told me all kinds of fantastic stories about his life: about the thirty-five-year-old daughter he had never known until last year, when she had tracked him down; about the beautiful prostitute in Switzerland whom he had brought to orgasm simply by talking dirty to her while she was sitting in a chair across from him, not even touching herself; about his near escape from a jealous husband who had chased him around the block with a butcher knife. His tales were a crazy brew. But he did say two things that I thought were very sensible and that I made a point of referring to later in life. The first was, "When you get to be my age, you realize that the only things you regret are the things you didn't do, not the things you did do." And the second was, "Women have civilized the world. If it weren't for women, men would live like wild beasts."

He talked so much that I often wondered whether the sex itself was secondary, merely a ploy to get me back to his apartment so that he could bombard me with his stories. I liked sleeping with him, although it was always a shock when he undressed; fully clothed he was a handsome, even a sexy man, but naked he stewed in old age. He would take a hold of his loose paunchy belly and swing it to one side so that he could penetrate me; I would shut my eyes and be grateful for the one or two Scotches I had drunk. Nevertheless, I must have been a little bit in love with him. He told me that many years ago he had published two detective novels that he had been very proud of. But he did not own any copies; they had been lost in a move, the books had gone out of print long ago. So one day I went to the public library, found his two novels, and stole them for him. I ruined my good library reputation for him. When I presented the books to him, he was touched; for a long time he simply turned them over and over in his hands, not saying a word.

Bart, the young graphic illustrator, was a very different sort of man than Alex. I liked him primarily because he was handsome, with thick clusters of curly blond hair, sly blue eyes, and a round, bantam chest. He was cheerful and embraced the universe of advertising without any irony at all; he could not understand why I was miserable and assured me that all I had to do was remain where I was and keep my bosses happy, and I would soon have everything I'd ever wanted in the world. "That's a great company. You're lucky to get in on the ground floor. It's going to grow bigger, too." When I mentioned to him that I had been toying with the idea of going back to graduate school he looked at me in horror and said, "But you'll be thirty by the time you get out." When I pointed out to him that I would be thirty in any case in that amount of time, he looked cold, as if I had said something that offended him. He was making a lot of money and he enjoyed buying himself things: an eight hundred dollar Burberry coat, a designer microwave, a brand new mint-green BMW. He never shopped for bargains; as he reasoned to me, "The more money I spend, the more money I'll have to make, and that'll force me to generate lots of business."

Bart liked me, but only up to a certain point. He was careful to let me know that there were other women in his life, such as the woman across the hall who constantly rang his doorbell on some flimsy excuse. He slyly insinuated that he would sometimes let her in. I was surprised at how hurt I was by these offhand remarks, in spite of the fact that I was well-supplied with extracurricular lovers myself. I must have been a little bit in love with him too—in fact, I was a little bit in love with all of them, and always just this little bit and never more. Something prevented me from taking anything but baby steps.

Bart was usually good company, light-hearted and fun-loving. But by accident one day I unearthed an unpleasant side to his nature. We were driving in his BMW—which he only drove outside of the city, because he was terrified of vandalism and scratches—and he remarked to me that a certain client of his had owed him money for a long time. "But of course he's a Jew," he said to me, "So what can you expect." I froze. He did not notice my discomfort. I could not bring myself to tell him that I was a Jew as well. Finally, many weeks later, I did tell him, and he was contrite and said, "Well, I know you're not *that kind* of a Jew."

I began to wonder, finally, what the hell I was doing with myself. I was so enveloped in the miasma of sexual chaos and workaday despair that my life had become, I could not see clearly. But one thing was certain, Ben: I was destroying myself, in a particularly masochistic and slow-acting way. After I had been with the advertising agency for a year, I began to request applications to various graduate programs for English literature. I did not know what else to do except to retrace my steps. Perhaps, if I could find my way back to the earnest, passionately committed student I had once been, there would be some hope for salvation. I could just as well have joined the army—the end result might have been equally beneficial, perhaps more so. But I was conventional and lacked imagination; school was what I did best, and so I pursued it.

When the applications arrived in the mail, I flipped at the pages with false bravado, but every time I tried to actually read the instructions, I got a violent headache, and I stuffed them under the pillow of my couch. But finally I began, inch by inch, to fill them out. I realized that completing the applications was an act of courage, a way of combating mortality and futility, and so I plodded forward with them as if my life depended on it. It took me three weeks to fill out the top portion of the first one, in which I was asked to reveal my name, address, phone number, date of birth, and the college I had attended.

Around the time that I was furtively contemplating a return to the world of academia, Alex surprised me by informing me one night over dinner that he had spoken to Jim and Bill and they had given him permission to assign me a direct mail piece. He leaned back in his chair and peered at me, narrowing his eyes, trying to gauge my reaction. He expected me to be pleased, and I was, at first. For a moment, even, my heart leaped, and I thought: at long last, salvation. I recognized the thud of hope. Perhaps this article would prove to be the hinge on which my future hung; perhaps, as Jim and Bill had insinuated, this past year had been my trial in purgatory, and I would soon be admitted to a higher circle of being. But these thoughts lasted no longer than the melting ice in Alex's highball. The experience of being Alex's lover, combined with the experience of working in the agency for a year, had turned me into a more cynical young woman. I had few hopes, and I understood that I must do everything required of me, even without hope. And so I accepted the copy writing assignment without comment, or complaint, or gratitude. I believe I surprised Alex by my unenthusiastic response. But he did not dwell on it; he was never daunted by my moods, he was too much in thrall to his own moods to be bothered much by mine.

The piece was to be a brochure for Ameritech's cellular phone, a device that was just beginning to emerge in the 1980s. Alex gave me the background I would need, as well as a lot of informational material from the company. He made a big speech about the assignment, strutting back and forth across his living room in his blue and white striped boxer shorts. "This is an enormous responsibility," he told me. "I am trusting you to deliver for me. I have, as you know, every faith in your innate ability and your native intelligence, but you're still an unknown factor. This is your chance to show Jim and Bill the stuff you're made of." I was at first shocked and then repulsed by his cliché-ridden pep talk. I had thought him better than that—wryer, with more of a jagged edge. It was only a two-page piece of print advertising, after all. And yet he was quite sincere; there was not a touch of irony in all his bombast. I could not take my eyes off his pendulous, pocked gray belly, and I prayed, Dear God, if I ever get out of this alive, I will never, ever sleep with an old man again, no, not if he were the only man left on earth.

I wrote the piece in a few hours the next night and brought it to Alex the morning after. I had not enjoyed writing it, but neither had I disliked writing it: it was a task, like sorting laundry or paying bills, something that had to be done. I did not find it particularly difficult to do. But Alex received my work with skepticism: he held the edge of my typewritten paper between thumb and forefinger and frowned and shook it slightly, as if to let the sediment fall to the bottom. Then he told me sternly that he would read it later and get back to me. As I was walking out of his office, he said, "Are you coming over tonight?"

So that night, it was the same thing again: Alex, weaving up and down the room in his underwear, holding my draft in his left hand, gesturing with his right; me, shivering in my green silk teddy on the edge of his leather couch, trying desperately to muster the right expression for the occasion—was it submissiveness informed by intelligence that was warranted? youthful awe? prideful nervousness? ambition masked by a desire to please? Or perhaps it was concupiscence that was really wanted. I was beginning to understand that Alex, being such a verbal man, found the process of revision to be an erotic experience.

"This is terrible," he told me. "I know you can do better than this. I can't even understand what you've written, so how would you expect some poor jerk who rips open his junk mail while he's sitting on the john to get the concept? You've got to grab them in the first second—no, in less than a second, in the first fraction of a second. You've got to *sell* the product, you've got to make it sexy. This—this is the most boring stuff I've ever read."

When I asked him if he could give me any concrete suggestions as to how I should revise the piece, he became irritated, and told me that was something I would have to arrive at myself. "Hard work. Hard, lonely work, young lady. You shouldn't even have to ask me such questions. I thought you called yourself a writer."

He was drunk—on Scotch, on words, on the invigorating role he was playing. And I was right about the concupiscence. I could not help noticing during his speech that he was terrifically aroused. I was soon divested of my green silk teddy, and we talked no more that evening.

The next night I spent more time revising my piece than I had spent writing it, and I agonized over it just a little more than I had the first time. I studied other direct mail pieces, trying to pick up some hints about how to be "sexy." By the time I was finished it was 2 A.M., and I was more than a little proud of myself.

But Alex tore the second version apart as well: tore it apart eloquently, then fucked me. And this went on for eight days and nights. I cursed Ameritech's cellular phone, which I could no longer even recognize as a phone after the hours and hours of rewrites. I rearranged paragraphs and rewrote paragraphs. I consulted a thesaurus, something I never did, and which was a sure sign that I had severely compromised myself. I began to ponder upon, God help me, *topic sentences.* I no longer trusted a word I had written, no, not even a comma or a semicolon, and I could certainly no longer remember why I was doing this, where this misguided ambition had originated.

And on the eighth night I could not bring myself to change a single word. I sat in front of my typewriter for an hour, drinking Ovaltine and eating Oreo cookies. The stinking piece sat there festering and I would not touch it. At ten o'clock I went to bed and slept soundly for the first time in a week.

The next day I presented Alex with my "revision." "Here," I told him. "This is the last time I'm doing this. Ever. I don't give a damn about the man sitting on the john reading his junk mail. Either you take it just the way it is, or you can do the job yourself, if you think you can do it better."

Approval registered on Alex's face; my rebelliousness pleased him. I could sense myself rising in his estimation: not just some hot young piece after all.

He read the draft with great excitement. "Now this," he said, his hand trembling, "is what I call writing. This will sell phones. This is what we were aiming for, during all those nights of hard work. I'm proud of you."

It was, of course, the exact same draft he had read two nights ago and attacked so savagely. I looked closely at him; his eyes were red, the blue irises swimming in blood. There were liver spots on his hands and wattles on his neck. And suddenly I began to feel sorry for him, so much so that tears came to my eyes. Old man, I'm getting out, I wanted to tell him, but you never will. The door is closed for you, but please forgive me if I slip through that crack, just wide enough for a girl. Don't hold it against me.

And I knew that he had once been handsome, young, and talented, and that he had been a real writer, had known what writing felt like, at least for a brief time.

When the Ameritech piece proved to be a success and generated many new orders for cellular phones, Jim and Bill were quite pleased with me. Jim introduced me to clients as "one of our potential new creatives." He winked and said, "In six months or so, as soon as we get it approved in the budget, I think you're going to have a new job description." At the weekly company meetings, many jokes were made about my newly discovered "talent." "So what would all your fancy professors think about this?" said Bill. Jim suggested that I arrange the minutes in sonnet form. "Throw in a couple of great metaphors for us, okay?" I knew that I had gone from being an upstart, slightly dangerous college girl to a feather in their cap. It was galling to think that they regarded me as their discovery, that they were gloating over the nimble management skills and daring corporate strategy that had enabled them to pluck me from the masses.

"What hillbillies they are," Alex remarked to me. "You'll soon be sailing way beyond them. Don't even bother being nice to those sorry specimens anymore. Just refuse to take their crap. People like us need people like that for a short time, but then we can dispense with them."

I saw so clearly now what had mystified me before: I was a pawn in Alex's epic revolutionary fantasy to tell the whole world to go fuck itself. It was a grand game he was playing. Hemmed in himself, able only to hobble uselessly one square sideways, he had recruited me as a classic front-runner. He would send me out into the open field primed for battle, armed to the teeth with the knowledge he himself had so painfully acquired over the years. Poor Alex. I saw I would be unable to ever forget him. I didn't know then if this unrelenting memory would be an asset or a liability in my future life, and I decided that only the passage of time could decide for me. Right then, I simply accepted the fact that he had gained an undeniable foothold in my consciousness. The fact was, the old man really did aim for me to succeed—he was not simply sacrificing me. He wanted me to be that rare thing, a winner. And then he wanted me to vomit it all back in their faces again. Fuck you, world. You're not worth the getting.

He both got what he wanted out of me and didn't get what he wanted: it's all a matter of context. I no longer had any desire to be a Junior Copy Writer, and my only problem now was how to disentangle myself with dignity. Quitting could only be interpreted as fear of success—which I certainly did have a fear of, although it was not becoming a Junior Copy Writer that frightened me. If I quit, Jim and Bill would hold me in contempt. They would soon write me off as a loser and an unexceptional human being. No, better imprint myself on them in some way. I would get myself fired. Bad behavior on my part would puzzle them, leave them guessing. Many years from now when they were old men, retired, drowning in deep leather chairs while sipping brandy in some downtown men's club, they'd remember me as a red blotch on their career. That was the way to go.

It was not hard getting fired: Alex had certainly goaded

me into subversion often enough that I was skilled in the techniques. I refused to type charts for them. I misfiled important papers and discreetly discarded others in the garbage can in Bart's office across the hall. I set up meetings with clients and told Jim and Bill the wrong time or the wrong place. I was rude to vice presidents on the phone. I batted my eyes at all salesmen who happened to wander off the elevator and ordered anything they cared to pitch to me, ramming giant holes in the quarterly budget. And all this in the name of initiative and ambition.

So it wasn't long before Jim and Bill sent Ellory to present me with a formal letter documenting all my misdeeds. Ellory's title was Account Manager, and to him fell all the tasks that Jim and Bill were too squeamish to perform themselves—firing freelancers and other staff, wrangling with the people in the budget office back in New York, and lying to clients about the status of projects, wheedling and negotiating for more time. The constant stress of having to be Jim and Bill's henchman had worn Ellory down; his hair was grizzled and sparse at the temples. He was kind-hearted. He hated having to take me in his office and read me the letter. "All you have to do, really, is apologize, that's all they want, and then everything will be status quo," he assured me. "Jim and Bill realize that this behavior is just—well, just an aberration for you. You've got a lot of potential; they don't want to lose you." Nervously he poked at his spectacles; his eyes pleaded silently with me to accept this offering, so that he would not have to execute the ultimate punishment. But I refused to apologize, and in a few more days, Ellory presented me with my dismissal. I packed my desk and left the advertising agency and never looked back.

But when I got home that afternoon, I found myself in no mood for celebration. My backside had been badly grazed by my narrow escape. How had it happened that I had mis-understood myself so profoundly? I had been treating my life as if it had been a circus act, with thrills and pratfalls: but there was no net to catch me, and the danger had proved quite real after all.

For me, there has always been something powerfully se-ductive about the misstep, the evasive act, the chance en-counter that leads to disorder and disintegration. And I have sometimes willed error into being. But a mistake that lasts a year of your life is no longer a mistake but a grievous transgression against your immortal soul.

And yet sometimes grace is offered. Often a limited grace, but even this is worth taking. A few weeks after my dishon-orable discharge, I received acceptances from both Cornell and the University of Michigan. I had worked in the adver-tising agency long enough to learn a thing or two, and so I called both English departments and told them I had also been accepted to the other school and had a dilemma about which one to choose. They both promptly offered me more money; the University of Michigan offered me a full fellow-ship, and so I said yes. In the autumn I would be returning to school.

I said goodbye to my lovers. Bart received the news with pleasant equanimity; he was already tiring of me. He took me out for a splendid dinner, made love to me even more splendidly, and told me to call him when I was home on spring break. (Over Christmas, he informed me, he'd be in Jamaica.)

The Greek gave me gifts. An expensive, butter-soft leather book bag, a gold-plated pen, a monogrammed ap-pointment book. I knew all this came out of the Bishop's pocket, but I was still touched. He told me that he would miss me very much, and to call him when I was home for Christmas break.

The Iranian-Jewish boy offered me his stoniest expression. His jaw seemed to harden into granite as I told him. Finally he said, "I hope you will finally find what you are looking for there. That you will not be disappointed. This year has been very despairing for you." I wrote down my new address and phone number for him and I said formally, "Please keep in touch."

Alex behaved badly, the worst of all. Although I knew that he was planning on marrying his long-standing mistress from Boston, he panicked and begged me to stay in Chicago. When I refused, he offered me five hundred dollars a month if I would continue to be his lover once I was in school, on the condition that I see him at least twice each month. I was tempted; for a poor graduate student, five hundred dollars is a lot of money. But I had started with him out of caprice, not calculation, and money was not what I had been after. Besides, the idea of myself as Alex's fancy woman did not jibe with my plans for asceticism, intellectual growth, and spiritual integrity. I turned him down.

Having made my farewells, I was off. I discovered that I was still limber, and capable of covering great distances on my own two feet.

Well, Benjamin, this is where I will stop. It is certainly not all I could tell you, but all letters are finite, and must end somewhere. You are no longer the two-and-a-half-year-old child you were when I began writing; now you are four, and that in itself is a humbling fact for your mother. To have written a hundred pages is one thing, but to have turned *four* and all which that signifies puts everything in a different perspective. Think of what an adult typically does within a year and a half, then think of what a child accomplishes between the ages of two-and-a-half and four. The fact that you have turned four is reason enough for me to stop: I can never hope to match that.

What will you make of my story? Writers are often dependent upon their readers for illumination, although it may seem as if the opposite is true, as if we are dispensing illumination. The truth is, we write blindly, creating light as we go along, and sometimes only a scant amount, just enough to see by, and precious little more. What we *hope* for is a different matter—order, coherence, veracity, supremacy over chaos and nothingness. And revenge, too. (That's the hardest one, since our wounds are often too abstract to avenge.) We can only be humbled by what we do achieve, and add our achievements to the collective efforts of our colleagues. The cumulative effect may come closer to approaching the ideal than anything we attempt individually. It *may*.

I fear that after reading my letter you may feel more frustrated than enlightened. Surely a thousand questions will spring to mind that I have not bothered to address, and you as the reader are probably entitled to your sense of indignation. I have left out things, there are serious gaps. Names, dates, years, even chronology—you are left scrambling for basic facts, and even after a most fastidious reading, you can barely piece anything together. Where was I born, how old were my parents, and where did they come from? What about my college years, why have I skipped over those? What hospital was I born in? What was the name of the suburb I grew up in, and who was my maternal grandmother? Why don't I talk more about my parents, your grandparents? What was going on in the world during my childhood and adolescence? (Why don't I mention Vietnam and the Cold War?) What was our household income, and what did my father do for a living? Did we own a car, and what make was it? Did I have a pet? I stated, in the beginning of this letter, that I wanted to present myself to you because I wanted you to know something about my history. But it is possible that I have turned myself into more of an enigma than I had intended. You may know less about the facts of my history now after having come to the end, than you knew at the beginning. You may even accuse me, at times, of deliberately throwing the wool over your eyes about certain events and time sequences.

Yet, on closer inspection, I see that something has emerged from these vignettes after all. The whole is possibly a tale about the birth of a writer, and it may also be a cautionary tale about the writing life—the devils of ego, isolation, doubt, social ineptitude, arrogance, loneliness, self-imposed misery, and failure that plague anybody who attempts it. And the power it confers, which is no delusion, and the first flush of awareness of that power. And the responsibility of bearing witness. I see also that I have written to you as a way of gaining the upperhand over fate: the Word trumps the Virus. The act of writing itself is, for me, part penitence and part celebration; I grieve for the errors I've made in my life, which writing only serves to uncover, and for the impossibility of ever rectifying them. Still, I permit myself to be triumphant, because in spite of all that folly and blindness, I have arrived here, at this late hour, to the very words I am at this moment typing on this page.

I see that my letter to you may also be about character, and the mysterious processes by which we become the people we were meant to be—or how we miss doing that and get diverted. My labors have had an unexpected and pleasurable byproduct: while excavating my character, I have also excavated yours. I foreshadow you. A certain rebelliousness that can have a petty motive at some times, a profound one at others; a lack of guile, and thus a frustrating

inability to obtain the things we need; a paradoxical tendency to be both too open-hearted and too withdrawn:
these are traits we both share. When you play one of your
"dinosaur games," taking your whole collection of meat-
eaters and plant-eaters into your room and acting out a
play that we are not allowed to watch, because you are
doing it only for yourself, I have the eerie sensation that
time has been compressed, that I am simultaneously myself,
your mother, fondly indulging your need for privacy, and
myself, a little girl, disappearing behind closed doors and
shutting out my own parents, who also stand guard for my
solitude.

You are not going to become an artist: happily, I can already tell from your behavior that this is not your natural
bent. But although you will manage to avoid the pitfalls of
an artistic temperament, nonetheless, I fear your path won't
be easy. Not with that quirky, rather fierce intelligence you
display and your often maniacal enthusiasms. You are con-
tentedly antisocial, pushing trains and trucks in your own
rhythm, not deeming it necessary to assimilate the rhythms
of other children. While you are occasionally attracted to
other children (usually older ones), you are not always sure
how to engage their attention, and usually resort to some
clownish display of crude gymnastics accompanied by a
child's version of punning and some innovative sound effects. You don't always win friends this way. I have heard of
other four year olds who invite each other home for play
dates, and insinuate themselves into some desirable company by offering up their favorite hook and ladder truck or
dispensing chocolates. You don't have this knack. When
ousted from a group because your overzealous bouncing
scatters all the blocks, you take it all in stride. When you
pulled the hair of a very grownup little girl in your pre-
school class, she flipped her tresses over the other shoulder

and announced, "Benjamin has *no* manners at all." This is true—your manners are primitive, and you don't yet understand why they are necessary, except to avoid rebuke. You don't especially *want* other children to like you. You are perfectly able to amuse yourself, and to concentrate on some solitary task without assistance from adults or children. In this respect you remind me so much of myself as a child that I don't know whether to rejoice at the similarities, as my vanity prompts me, or to be fearful, as my maternal instincts advise.

I hope after reading this letter that you will be able to divine something about who I was before your advent in my life, and how I came to be the person I am today. You might recognize the child in the mother you know, or you may be able to reconstruct the mother from the child. Connections that you might not have made if this letter did not exist will possibly be facilitated. Certain facets of my personality might begin to make more sense. There is a wonderful children's book called *Are You My Mother?* in which a newly hatched bird whose mother has gone off in search of food tumbles out of the nest and asks every being or thing he encounters if it is his mother. He meets a cow, a dog, a cat, an old truck, a steam shovel. He hopes, he yearns—but with each he is disappointed. They are *not* his mother. When will he find her? He begins to despair. Finally, he returns to his nest and his mother appears, worm in mouth. His joy is immense—the long search and the many setbacks were all worthwhile because in the end he has learned to distinguish between his mother and the rest of the world. And so the baby bird's survival is ensured. It is my hope that after reading this letter you will be able to recognize a steam shovel for what it is, and your mother for what she is. You will be able to claim me immediately, without having to undergo the baby bird's blind and agonizing journey. If you are able to claim me, then this letter has been a success.

Darling Benjamin, you are already beginning to have stories to tell about your own life and my dearest wish is that I will be there to listen to even more of them, or to play my part, if that's what's called for, even in the most marginal way. The important thing is that they are *yours* and only you can present them in the manner in which you most desire them to be presented; you hold the power over your stories. Remember this.

All your most significant work is ahead of you, as far as the building of your character is concerned. And it's *your* work. The foundation has been laid, and your fond parents have tried to ensure that you have the best possible materials to build with and we like to believe that we have offered you some kind of useful guidance, a blueprint. But beyond the foundation, think of all that needs to be done—the walls built brick by brick, each brick representing a new experience, a new human being; the roof of ethics, often leaky, and in constant need of repair; the tangle of wiring and pipes, those conduits of opinions, inferences, insults, judgments, desires, grievances, all in constant danger of becoming scrambled; the insulation (always love, in my system of metaphors); the windows—clarity, epiphany— and as far as the decor, all the playful embellishments, then the paring down. And the pillars and beams of self-knowledge supporting it all.

I believe firmly that the most important task we have in life is to unmask ourselves, so that we will eventually discover what our lives mean to us, and what it is we are meant to love. I wish you luck with this task, Benjamin!

Your loving Mother

Notes

On page 56 I quote a passage from *The Remembrance of Things Past, Swann's Way*, by Marcel Proust (translated from the French by C. K. Scott Moncrieff, Vintage Books edition, 1970). The passage is in the chapter entitled "Swann in Love," on page 289.

The statistics cited on pages 70–71 are from the HIV/AIDS Surveillance Report, "U.S. HIV and AIDS cases reported through December 1999," Year-end edition Vol. 11, No. 2. Specifically, I refer to the Commentary on page 5 and to Table 7, on page 16, "AIDS cases by sex, age at diagnosis, and race/ethnicity, reported through December, 1999, United States." The Report is published by the Centers for Disease Control and Prevention in Atlanta, Georgia. I also refer to two websites offering international statistics: www.WHO.org and www.cdc.gov/HIV.

I quote a poem by Yeats, "When You Are Old," in its entirety on page 214. This is from *The Collected Poems of W. B. Yeats*, Revised Second Edition, edited by Richard J. Finneran (New York: Scribner, 1996).

Acknowledgments

I would like to thank Thomas Mallon for the wise words and invaluable suggestions he offered during the process of editing and revising, and for his warm support in general. Thanks are also due to my long-suffering husband, Griff Butler, who puts up with having a writer in the house; to my mother, Ethel Peterson, an unflagging source of love and support; and to Deborah Kahn, Jay Butterman, Roslyn Banish, and Mary Rose McCudden.